# WHERE IT HURTS

## Dispatches *from the* Emotional Frontlines *of* Medicine

**Edited by**
**DONNA BULSECO**
Foreword by Rita Charon, MD

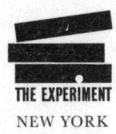

THE EXPERIMENT
NEW YORK

WHERE IT HURTS: *Dispatches from the Emotional Frontlines of Medicine*
Copyright © 2026 by Donna Bulseco
Foreword copyright © 2026 by Rita Charon

All rights reserved. Except for brief passages quoted in newspaper, magazine, radio, television, or online reviews, no portion of this book may be reproduced, distributed, or transmitted in any form or by any means, electronic or mechanical, including photocopying, recording, or information storage or retrieval system, without the prior written permission of the publisher.

The Experiment, LLC
220 East 23rd Street, Suite 600
New York, NY 10010-4658
theexperimentpublishing.com

THE EXPERIMENT and its colophon are registered trademarks of The Experiment, LLC. Many of the designations used by manufacturers and sellers to distinguish their products are claimed as trademarks. Where those designations appear in this book and The Experiment was aware of a trademark claim, the designations have been capitalized.

The Experiment's books are available at special discounts when purchased in bulk for premiums and sales promotions as well as for fundraising or educational use. For details, contact us at info@theexperimentpublishing.com.

Library of Congress Cataloging-in-Publication Data available upon request

ISBN 979-8-89303-104-1
Ebook ISBN 979-8-89303-105-8

Cover and text design by Beth Bugler
Cover illustration by Mohamed Mahfouz Sylla

Manufactured in the United States of America

First printing March 2026
10 9 8 7 6 5 4 3 2 1

The authorized representative in the EU for product safety and compliance is Easy Access System Europe, Mustamäe tee 50, 10621 Tallinn, Estonia easproject.com | gpsr.requests@easproject.com.

# Acclaim for *Where It Hurts*

"I'll not soon forget the voices of these dedicated physicians, nurses, teachers, and technicians who treat their patients with humanity, compassion, and humility. I was riveted and moved by this collection."
—**Wally Lamb,** #1 *New York Times*–bestselling author of *She's Come Undone* and *The River Is Waiting*

"A powerful anthology with its origins in caregiving, and the pain and suffering that invokes it. The humanity of these poems, stories, and essays makes for compelling reading, an opportunity for spiritual enlargement, and a reminder of why medicine is so much more than service."
—**Thomas McGuane,** author of *A Wooded Shore* and *The Longest Silence*

"The honest, heartbreaking, and uplifting voices of doctors and nurses, EMTs and medical students not only bring us behind the scenes of surgeries and intubations and autopsies, but also let us into their hearts and minds. This book will continue to echo long after you finish it."
—**Ann Hood,** bestselling author of *The Knitting Circle* and *Comfort: A Journey Through Grief*

"Ranging panoramically in perspective and tone . . . this collection offers readers grand works of literature in miniature. Each piece is a perfect morsel of perception: a window into the soul of a caregiver and a mirror for the reader's reflection. A testament to the power of narrative medicine, *Where It Hurts* belongs on every healer's nightstand."
—**Jacob M. Appel, MD,** author of *Who Says You're Dead?*

"*Where It Hurts* gathers voices from the intimate, vital space between clinicians and patients, tracing the invisible threads that connect body and story. Tender, raw, and deeply human."—**Danielle Ofri, MD, PhD,** author of *What Doctors Feel* and editor in chief of *Bellevue Literary Review*

"Gritty and abrasive. Brutally honest and forged with sweat equity and spilled blood. *Where It Hurts* is a collection of essays and poems that will seize your heart. Even when I wanted to retreat and calm my soul, I kept turning the pages."—**Wes Ely, MD,** physician-scientist and practicing intensivist at Vanderbilt University, and author of *Every Deep-Drawn Breath*

"*Where It Hurts* cuts to the core of what it means to be a clinician today."—**Sneha Mantri, MD,** director of medical humanities at Duke University School of Medicine

"Masterfully spotlights the humanity, humility, and vulnerability of clinicians at the front lines of health care in the United States. Their candid stories offer a window into the messy, poignant, and meaningful facets of the human condition."—**Erica C. Kaye, MD,** oncologist at St. Jude Children's Research Hospital

"A healing balm for anyone impacted by their own or someone else's illness—which is to say anyone who is human."—**Elizabeth Lahti, MD,** associate professor and director of narrative medicine at Oregon Health & Science University School of Medicine

"*Where It Hurts* lifts the curtain on the hidden dramas of medicine. A must-read for anyone going into a health care profession, or anyone who may need their services."—**Randi Hutter Epstein, MD,** writer in residence and director of the Writing for the Public program at Yale University School of Medicine

"This rich, compelling collection will help physicians, nurses, and their patients . . . learn important lessons about human nature and what it means to care for each other."—**Joel Howell, MD, PhD,** director emeritus of the Medical Arts Program, University of Michigan Medical School

"Remarkable and varied. This is a book for clinicians, educators, and anyone drawn to ponder this enterprise of living in our beautiful, perfectly imperfect bodies."—**Deepu Gowda, MD,** assistant dean for medical education, Kaiser Permanente Bernard J. Tyson School of Medicine

"Wise, tender, funny, and vulnerable."—**Jay Baruch, MD,** author of *Tornado of Life: A Doctor's Journey through Creativity and Constraints in the ER*

"An extraordinary collection that highlights the intersection between medical mysteries and the mysteries of the human spirit. Each piece is provocative, inspiring, resonant, humane. A book to return to over and again for insight, compassion, and courage."—**Lou Ann Walker,** editor in chief of *The Southampton Review*

"This book should be required reading for students, physicians, nurses, and anyone who has to deal with the health care system (and that includes all of us!). Highly recommended."—**David G. Thoele, MD, and Marjorie Getz, PhD,** codirectors of the narrative medicine program at Advocate Health

*For the shining stars in my constellation:*
*Dana, Roy, and Veradonna*

# Contents

Foreword: The Healing Powers of Narrative, *Rita Charon*  1
A World Writ Large: The Rewards of Real Stories, *Donna Bulseco*  5

**1    WRANGLING DRAGONS: Self-Doubt**
  Your First Pediatric Intubation, *Rachel Kowalsky*  12
  Newbie, *Elizabeth Osmond*  15
  Polychroma, *Justin Millan*  17
  Things I Learned from Pole Dancing That
     I Did Not Learn from Residency, *Elise Mullan*  23
  Coming Out of the Medical Closet, *Angelica Recierdo*  28
  Becoming a Doctor, *Brent Schnipke*  31
  Getting to Know Dying, *Anna Belc*  34
  Night Watch, *Dana Gage*  38
  Body of Work, *Anna Dovre*  42

**2    A THIN LINE: Love and Hate**
  Pretending Not to Know, *Priscilla Mainardi*  50
  Love, Frank, *Cheryl Bailey*  55
  Yours, *Nina Gaby*  61
  My Favorite Patient, *Sarah Harvin*  65
  Untarnished, *Ali Rizvi*  67
  Bruised Apples, *Jack Coulehan*  73
  Dr. Ortega and the Fajita Man, *Richard B. Weinberg*  79

**3  THE SOUND AND THE FURIES: Shame and Anger**
Old Scrubs, *Bruce H. Campbell*   86
Black Tango, *Philip Berry*   90
Kübler-Ross, *S. K. Rancy*   94
The Halo, *Xi Chen*   96
Intro to Physicianship, *Lala Tanmoy Das*   102
Red Line Rising, *Michael Brown*   104
What Does a Medical Student Do All Day? *Maya J. Sorini*   110
D/D, *Maureen Hirthler*   112
Chronic Black Excellence, *Michael Arnold*   114
Managed Care, *Jennifer Anderson*   117

**4  LOST IN TRANSLATION: Confusion**
Ambulance Stories, *B. Shepard Blue*   124
The Spaces Between, *Jennifer Li*   132
When Suicide Speaks Arabic, *Ibrahim Sablaban*   136
Across the Great Rift, *Sophia Gauthier*   141
It's Not That, *Katherine Flores Guzman*   148
Vicious, *Tim Cunningham*   150

**5  ALONE AGAIN, UNNATURALLY: Loneliness and Loss**
Being Seen, *Cara Haberman*   156
Infectious, *Doug Hester*   159
Harvest, *William Bachman*   161
Late, *I. Cori Baill*   165
The Doctor's White Room, *Sumit Parikh*   168
Invisible, *Joanne Wilkinson*   170
Calluses, *Laura B. Vater*   173
The Idea of Him, *H. Reade Joo*   177

## 6   THE PLAGUE YEARS: Fear and Panic

The Shape of the Shore, *Rana Awdish*   182
My First Mask Was a White Coat, *Lauren Fields*   190
Everything, *Simone Blaser*   192
Where Are You, Mary Oliver? *Katharine Lawrence*   197
Resuscitation, *Daly Walker*   199
Curveballs, *Kaitlyn Reasoner*   206

## 7   DEATH SENTENCES: Feeling Mortal

Teatime, *Catherine Read*   212
Omens, *Ryan Boyland*   215
Cause of Death, *Yu Li*   218
No Word, *E. E. Toksu*   225
The Boxer, *Aniqa Azim*   230
To Pronounce, *Thomas J. Doyle*   233
Haglund's Deformity, *Elizabeth Lanphier*   237
First Will and Testament, *Anna Stacy*   239

## 8   THE WONDER YEARS: Curiosity and Tenderness

Letter to a 93-Year-Old Cadaver Who Died
    from Multiple Causes, *Jennifer Stella*   244
A Shot of Perspective, *Jordana Kritzer*   247
For the Old Man Buying a Stuffed Giraffe, *Ben Goldenberg*   252
A Tale of Three Breasts, *Carol Scott-Conner*   255
Top Surgery, *Angela Tang-Tan*   259
Beethoven Symphony No. 5, *Mitali Chaudhary*   264
Beholding Something Fine, *Laura Johnsrude*   267
Stroppy Sevens, *Trisha Paul*   272

Acknowledgments   273
About the Editor   278

FOREWORD

# The Healing Powers of Narrative

RITA CHARON

NARRATIVE PRACTICES ILLUMINATE lives lived amid illness with meaning, with movement, with moments of being. Sometimes hidden, always mysterious, simultaneously understood and misunderstood, illness interrupts the no-illness with an alternative and defining reality. It can barge in violently or sidle in softly, either stealing the before-illness life or accompanying it. Professional caregivers have names for illnesses: acute, chronic, diagnosable, idiopathic, contagious, psychogenic, curable, terminal. Patients and their families come to know the character of the illness: night-stalking, wakefulness-sapping, fleeting, needy, greedy, gruesome. In its wake they become sorrowful, anxious, courageous, impatient, indomitable, adaptable, resigned, triumphant. They can become other persons altogether or become all the more deeply themselves.

All of these dimensions of illness emerge from the stories of *Where It Hurts*. We readers receive authentic portraits of the patients and of the clinicians and trainees who care for them. From a first-year medical student stunned at what she's chosen to do with her life to a nurse who must care for a murderer on her hospital unit, the voices of these essays and stories and poems bring us the emotional shock and moral challenge of their work. As we read, we are prompted to self-examination. We wonder: *What would I do?* and we learn from the insight of the writers. The forms vary from metered poetry to fragmented post-modern verse, from short fiction to memoir to in-the-moment reportage. A poetic self-declaration overcomes the barrage of self-doubt as a Black physician comes to terms with racist insinuations that surround him. A poignant short story depicts an aging surgeon who must doubt his fitness to continue his beloved work. A raw display of clinicians' lives in the early days of COVID-19 reminds the reader of the horrors of the pandemic and the sacrifices of health professionals, some of whom perished in the plague they were battling.

These creative works are manifestations of the sub-discipline of health humanities called narrative medicine. In the early 2000s, I convened a group of clinicians and humanities scholars at Columbia University to recognize the power of reading and writing and immersion in works of art in the care of the sick. We called our work "narrative medicine" to remind others that illnesses have stories to tell and that clinicians can learn to hear them. Despite the challenges of clinical work, health professionals can deepen their own capacity to recognize what they, their patients, and their patients' families experience. In the journal *Intima*, from which the pieces in this book have been reprinted, doctors and nurses and social workers publish their heartful memoirs of triumphs and losses, sharing their own journeys of healing. They open themselves to the mysteries of illness that, unlike sacramental or religious phenomena, arise on this earth, in ordinary settings of daily life, to deepen their own sense of the holy. The more clearly and generously these caregivers attend to what their patients go through and the more attentive they become to their own fears and hopes, the more powerful is the care they can give.

Columbia's narrative medicine has spread to many health care sites in the United States and abroad. Among the field's more lasting contributions are perhaps the therapeutic uses to which narrative medicine has been put. At Columbia, adult palliative care clinicians meet monthly with a literary scholar and writing coach to better understand patients' and their families' experiences at the end of life. The Eating Disorders Clinic at Columbia Psychiatry has brought writing skills to the adolescent patients struggling with life-threatening body image distortions. These narrative interventions are shown to improve patients' well-being and clinicians' insight and satisfaction with their work.

I have known and worked with Donna Bulseco and her co-editors at *Intima: A Journal of Narrative Medicine*, for years. Brilliant writers and editors, all trained in the Master of Science in Narrative Medicine graduate program at Columbia, they curate and propagate the central values and methods of our field. They advance our deepest principles by soliciting work from those who stand at the frontlines of medicine. I feel proud and humble to see this magnificent collection of works, chosen with aesthetic and clinical sensibility, emerge from our young tradition of narrative medicine. Clinical readers will become better nurses and doctors and social workers for witnessing what these stories divulge. Patients and families will come to understand their own battles with ill health with the inspiration and meaning-making of *Intima*'s offerings. Fellow mortals all, in sharing our stories we enrich one another with wisdom, with knowledge, and with the words that beckon us into relation.

---

**RITA CHARON** is a general internist and literary scholar and one of the founders of the field of narrative medicine. She completed her MD at Harvard Medical School and her PhD in English at Columbia University. She is the Bernard Schoenberg Professor of Social Medicine, Professor of Medicine, and founding chair of the Department of Medical Humanities and Ethics at Columbia's Vagelos College of Physicians & Surgeons. Her research in narrative medicine has been supported by the National Institutes of Health (NIH), the National Endowment for the Humanities (NEH), and many private foundations. She has authored, co-authored, or co-edited four books on narrative medicine. The NEH, the NIH, the Association of American Medical Colleges, and numerous medical associations have honored her with awards and distinctions. She lectures and teaches internationally and publishes extensively in leading medical and literary journals, including the *New England Journal of Medicine*, *Lancet*, *Journal of the American Medical Association*, *Academic Medicine*, *Narrative*, *Henry James Review*, *Poetics Today*, and *SubStance*.

# A World Writ Large: The Rewards of Real Stories

DONNA BULSECO

As we've seen time and again in medical dramas, from *St. Elsewhere* to *The Pitt*, stories about medicine call forth the deep emotions we all experience, from self-doubt, anger, and love to hatred, panic, curiosity, shame, and wonder. The essays, poems, and short stories in this collection, all drawn from *Intima: A Journal of Narrative Medicine*, tap into these universal emotions and provide insight into ourselves and others, in sickness and in health. These are urgent tales from doctors, nurses, social workers, EMTs, psychiatrists, and other caregivers. They invite us into real places—emergency rooms, surgical theaters, examination rooms, and morgues—to witness their work through their eyes and their words and to recognize our common strengths and vulnerabilities.

The origin of *Intima*, and by extension *Where It Hurts*, begins with a new model of health care called "narrative medicine," a discipline created at Columbia University in 2000 by the visionary internist Rita Charon and a group of fellow scholars of film, philosophy, art, and social justice. Narrative medicine uses great works of literature and art to teach doctors, nurses, patients, caregivers, and essential workers how to read, listen, interpret, and respond to stories about health and illness. With narrative medicine, Dr. Charon brought an intelligent empathy to the world of medicine.

Out of this movement and the outpouring of narratives from students in Columbia's Narrative Medicine program, *Intima* began to take shape in May and June of 2011, and the inaugural issue was published in the fall. The founding editors codified *Intima*'s mission to enhance empathy and understanding between caregivers and patients by publishing soul-searching stories, essays, and poetry. The ability to reflect on the world and on ourselves provides truth and meaning for all of us, and it's an essential component of the works in *Where It Hurts*. Indeed, the idea of the "epiphany" informs much of the work in this collection, thanks to the emphasis on it by Mario de la Cruz, a founding editor of *Intima*, who remains an inspiring member of its editorial board today.

An astonishing array of clinical tales form the basis of *Where It Hurts*, grouped into chapters organized by emotion. Chapter 1, for instance, is titled "Wrangling Dragons: Self-Doubt" and takes its name from a line in "Your First Pediatric Intubation," a short story by an ER physician whose checklist to get through a difficult task includes: "First, eat a meal. Then kick your dragons to the curb. The dragons of your self-doubt, my dear! You rode them all the way here." The essay "Things I Learned from Pole Dancing That I Did Not Learn from Residency," which was given an honorable mention in *Best American Essays 2023*, edited by Vivian Gornick, speaks honestly about living up to high expectations. Poems like "Becoming a Doctor" hit close to the bone, describing the fraught physical and mental challenges of doctoring.

A later chapter, "Lost in Translation: Confusion," addresses the unease often brought about by cultural clashes and gender differences in essays like "When Suicide Speaks Arabic," an intriguing look at conversations that fail to communicate. "Alone Again, Unnaturally: Loneliness and Loss" is a chapter about the inevitability of solitude, in medicine and in life, while the essays and poems in "The Plague Years: Fear and Panic" lay out the fearful effects of the COVID-19 crisis on patients, clinicians, and the world. A standout is the essay "The Shape of the Shore" by Rana Awdish, a critical care doctor. It was honored in 2020 with the Sidney Award, given annually by David Brooks, an opinion columnist for *The New York Times*, for outstanding long-form essays. Two final chapters reflect on mortality ("Death Sentences: Feeling Mortal") and happiness ("The Wonder Years: Curiosity and Tenderness").

Our journal's name, *Intima*, has a specific resonance for us. Narrative involves the intimate connection between people who yield and gain from the experience of sharing stories. The word *intima* refers to the lining of blood vessels, which speed blood to the heart and brain, an apt metaphor for narratives that speak to the emotions and the intellect. The title of *Where It Hurts* is likewise an acknowledgment of the intimacy and vulnerability of sharing our stories and the emotional and intellectual value of engaging with the medical world, a place where living and dying—and all of the feelings in between—come into play. The narratives collected in *Where It Hurts* appeal to our hearts and minds and, we hope, will speed connections between those providing care and those receiving it, making healing a common goal for everyone.

# WHERE IT HURTS

# 1

# WRANGLING DRAGONS

*Self-Doubt*

SHORT STORY

# Your First Pediatric Intubation

RACHEL KOWALSKY

FIRST, EAT A meal. Then kick your dragons to the curb. The dragons of your self-doubt, my dear! You rode them all the way here. Have you read the chapter? That will help. Let's go.

**1. Dress in a plastic gown.** Gather your endotracheal tube, laryngoscope, suction, stylet, syringe, pink tape. Connect the child to the monitor, the IV to its tubing, face mask to blue bag. Ask for medications early, and dose with care. Never do math in your head.

**2. Take your place as per the diagram.** You at the head, team leader at the foot, nurses to left and right. Chest compressor at the chest, of course, and hope that you won't need it. Tech there, clerk there, X-ray here then there, scribe, pharmacist, parents. You're in a circle of people; at its center, one child. You can process this later. Or now. You can process it now. Bright room, many people, small child. Okay, that's enough.

**3. Position the airway.** Lift the child, slide a towel beneath the shoulders. Ease the head back, chin up, good. Now the airway is ready, sleek and straight as a tunnel. Don't cut off the clothes;

this is not a television show. Ease them off and hand them to the mother—unless they are bloody, then cut them.

**4. Preoxygenate.** This buys you time in later steps. Push air through the tunnel to the lungs. Consider your career choice, and what tunnels are for: shelter, escape, crossing. I crossed too. Story, body, ocean, grief—to get here. Flew in on the back of a dragon.

**5. Maintain situational awareness.** You now stand in a circle of love. It's an awful cliché, but allowed in this context—life and death—another trope we invoke all day. Don't worry too much about all this, the time-worn language, the circle, mortality. You're just the airway person.

**6. Write love letters.** On the walls of the room, the back of scrub caps, the Breslow measuring tape. Take the mother's hand, draw her closer. Watch for dragons in the corners of the room.

**7. Wrangle dragons.** I'm sorry to say the dragons are here, those minstrels of your obstinate self-doubt. They've been exorcised, banished, left for dead at the side of the road, but this room, the trauma bay, is their last stronghold. Their silver and green scales are stunning, but don't look. Don't think about the boys on the bus, the filthy song they sang, or the one who scorned your love. Blow up the song in your mind. This room is a speck on a turtle's back. Think of the loves you have known.

**8. Speak loudly and clearly.** *Nurses, doctors, faithful pharmacist, we are going to sedate now.* Tell the scribe too. It's a wonderful word, scribe. A listener with a plume in hand, paid to bear witness and write it all down. Where did this story begin?

**9. Focus despite the ghosts who haunt your circle.** Noah's sister, Inez's son, Sara's ex. They all hover at elbows and hang on shoulders, it's a problem. Remember when we talked about (sorry) love? Send some to Noah, Inez, Sara, and obviously the scribe. Ghosts may only speak when spoken to, so don't do that. The room is crowded now between the people, the dragons, and the ghosts. Focus.

10. **Pass your scope, lift it up, behold the illumined airway.** The white V of the vocal cords pops into view. Relax, smile, tell a joke. Dragons hate jokes, they cringe and sulk in their corners. Pass the tube through the cords. Tape it in place with the pink tape. It's got to be pink, I don't know why. You're full of questions. Listen for breath sounds.

You thought you were done, but it's tricky— such stories don't have endings. Choose another beginning, like wheeling your patient to the ICU. The ghosts will follow, you know that much. The dragons will try, but they're too large to exit the room. They live there, in the trauma bay. Like you, they have the inconvenience of a body. The blessing and the agony of a body.

---

**RACHEL KOWALSKY** is a first-generation Guatemalan American writer and pediatric emergency physician in New York City. She is also a four-time Pushcart Prize nominee and winner of the inaugural *New England Journal of Medicine* short story prize. Learn more about her work at rachelkowalskymd.com.

# Newbie

ELIZABETH OSMOND

*After Caroline Bird*

You thought you could cannulate a vein, but it turns out
you were just putting a key in a lock. And that wasn't a night
shift you worked, it was staying up 'til the wee hours at
Glastonbury festival. And that wasn't an electronic discharge
summary you typed, you were tapping out a bad version of
"Rocket Man" on the piano. What if you thought you could
prescribe an opiate but instead you had just written
a smutty note? And that ward round presentation where
you remembered *all* the signs and symptoms of systemic lupus?
A rambling story in the pub. You thought that you intubated
a difficult airway when in fact you applied your eyeliner
in a dark smudge with all the medical students looking on.
Then you put your laptop safely in the fridge
called the consultant "mum"
put a kiss at the end of the handover text
all the while nodding to yourself like

"yeah, this is how it's done"
while dropping the bleep down the toilet

---

**ELIZABETH OSMOND** is a neonatal consultant in the United Kingdom. She writes poetry as a form of reflective practice, and her work has been published in many literary journals and anthologies. She is working on her first poetry collection. Find her on Bluesky at @bethosmond.bsky.social.

# Polychroma

## JUSTIN MILLAN

We sit opposite each other, my six-year-old daughter and I. She is the artist, I am the model. From my position across the table I can see her rendition of me, upside down. She has outlined my head with pencil. Now she surveys the crayons. "Should I use peach for your skin?" she says.

"Only if I'm healthy," I mutter.

"What?"

Complexion fluctuates, sometimes subtly, sometimes broadly. Our skin color is not a constant: it is a metric, prone to volatility, that presents the most elemental of changes to the exterior world.

One evening, my ambulance was summoned to a little brick house on the edge of the woods.

The subject was an elderly man, bent over the sofa's edge, ribs heaving, gulping air with all his might, while his wife nervously zigzagged around the room. The distress was early, and he still had the red-faced look of someone who is overexerting himself. We snapped an oxygen mask on his head, then, through a combination of guiding and lifting, relocated him onto the stretcher.

There was no path between the house and the back of the ambulance, only uneven earth, rock-pitted, that wrenched the stretcher this way and that. His color changed. Something siphoned away that hot, crimson shade; in its vacancy, his head took on a kind of gray glow, as if he were in the very early stages of morphing into a concrete statue. He's done too much, I realized. Even though we labored to move the stretcher while he rode above us like some enfeebled king, the bumpy ride forced him to stabilize his trunk. Each exertion was like another puncture in an ever-deflating tire—and now he was driving on the rim.

In the ambulance, we tried nebulized albuterol. He deteriorated. He was staring at me over the irregular dome of the mask. The little red numbers on the oximeter dipped to 60 percent. My captain flipped open the protocol book to the dyspnea section. "Ah. It *is* terbutaline," he said calmly. "I thought that came next, but I wasn't sure."

He placed the bored needle tip under the hairy skin on the man's arm and squeezed the syringe. For an interval, there was no discernible effect. Then, it came—a kind of solidity to his respirations, manifested by an ever-growing delay between gasps. "He's coming around," my captain said. The oximeter numbers leapt into the '80s. I grabbed a pen and the metal clipboard. When I turned to look at him again, a salmon color had spread across his forehead.

Soon, the salmon warmed toward rose red. Not some florist's rose on Valentine's Day, but a faded rose, long dead, desiccated, destemmed, and blown about by autumn winds. Still, I would take it. It was the red of heat, blood, and life overall, where before there had been only stone.

～

When I teach my children to color, I encourage them to use a lot of different crayons for flesh.

"Skin is not just brown, or peach. It's a mix," I say. Together, we study our arms under natural light.

"I see white, gray, blue, yellow, pinks, browns."

Crayons make it easy. With a light touch, the wax blends into a soft mash, just as in healthy skin the melanin, carotene, vascular beds, and other tissues commingle. But push too hard, and one color will dominate abnormally.

I worked at a facility where we accepted patients with liver failure. These people often had yellow skin due to their bodies' inability to clear bilirubin. One evening, I was the admitting nurse for one of these yellowed people, a young woman who rolled in from an ICU. Alcoholism had pushed her into multi-organ failure. She was on life support. She had ascites, an abnormal buildup of fluid in the abdomen; her checkered gown bulged grotesquely at the midsection.

She was delirious. I put her in mitts to keep her from tearing out her tracheostomy, as well as to protect the staff from her onslaughts. Her agitation became the center of the admission. I still have a vivid memory of her yellow face contorted in rage as she battered me with the mitts. Nothing held her back—not the tether of the ventilator, not her obvious deconditioning, not her engorged belly, which was nearly as large as a third-trimester pregnancy.

Toward the end of my shift, aides washed her while I stood in the doorway giving a report to the night nurse. I was relieved to get rid of her, but now, when I looked over at her, I felt pity. The room was dark except for the halogen fixture over the bed. It was hard to see the yellow flesh in this light. The scene reminded me of an old Renaissance painting, where the focal point is illuminated and the periphery is in darkness. The aides had the bed flat and they had stripped away her gown and undone the restraints. She was limp, no fight in her, and her thin, atrophied extremities trembled. One of the aides wrang a wet towel out over her body. The soapy water cascaded down her bulbous abdomen, each of the suds twinkling like a tiny crystal.

―

Hands and feet, when illustrated by beginning artists like my children, can often take on a demented look. I find that they struggle to angle the pencil tip so it generates a fine line. As a result, a chunky dark stripe borders the extremity. Digits become black claws.

I cared for a young man whose left foot terminated in a row of necrotic toes. The right foot had already been chopped down to the arch. Diabetes, peripheral vascular disease, obesity, trauma, noncompliance—the "at fault" list was a mosaic. He ambulated by donning large foam boots and leaning on a cane.

Care for these wounds was relatively simple. After all, the damage was already done: the nerves were extinguished and the tissue was charcoal.

He was frank about his health problems, so one day, as I crouched on the floor, wiping those hard, crusty black toes with betadine, I said, "When I take off the dressings, and you see your toes like this, what do you think? How does it make you feel?"

"Eh," he said. He turned away from his tablet and looked down at his foot, which was cradled in my gloved hands. He shrugged and returned his attention to the screen, "I'm used to it."

---

Sometimes, when drawing with my children, I fill in the characters with stripes, spots, and zigzags. It's just for fun, a way to spice up the image and perhaps provoke their curiosity.

Yet it is not all fantasy.

When I was a new nurse, I encountered a horrific case that haunts me to this day. A man was admitted for a six-week regimen of intravenous antibiotics. Outwardly, he appeared unafflicted. He had black hair trimmed into a crewcut and a large round nose. His intellect was severely limited by a congenital condition. He could follow only simple commands.

After the first week, problems developed. It started with a macular rash on his torso. While I don't recall the exact characteristics of the lesions, I remember my general impression, which was that he'd become spotted. And, although he couldn't verbalize the sensation, pruritus was obvious. We treated it with an anti-itch lotion, fed him antihistamine tablets in apple sauce, and changed the antibiotic. The lotion was white; it made pastel discs out of the lesions.

Over the next few days, the situation degenerated. The rash expanded to his back, groin, and extremities. Each sprouting of a new lesion severely altered the ratio of rash-skin to unblemished skin; he was effectively turning red. Staff who didn't know him, who were passing by the room and seeing him from the corner of their eye, would halt and do a double-take.

Other manifestations followed, including precipitously high fevers. The order came to use a cooling blanket. This involved placing a thermal probe in his rectum, then forcing him to lie on a vinyl pad that was supplied with ice-cold water from a machine.

My means to soothe this man were limited. Antipyretics and analgesics seemed to do nothing. He became anorectic. As his body's thermal set point shifted this way and that, chills racked his body. He toiled atop the pad, emitting plaintive groans, with only a thin sheet over him for comfort.

Understandably, in this state, given the pruritus, fevers, and the cooling blanket, he could not sleep. Even our life-support patients, who often appeared to be some of the most wretched souls on earth, would typically rest a little bit each day. This man had no respite. None. And because of his intellectual disability, try as I did, I could not make him understand what was going on.

I paced at the bedside. Charting on him, I felt at a loss as to what to write. I was powerless. It rattled me.

I tended to visualize pain and adversity as troughs, chasms, or holes, but this man's misery was low beyond low. It was so low, it went high, an inversion of all the anguish I'd yet seen. It was an apex of suffering that cast a hard shadow on all of my work. It still does.

―

My daughter dashes at the chin to evoke my scraggly beard. She has drawn my lips as a lavender block. The size and shape of the eyes are a mismatch, but the stare is equal: straight ahead, unemotional.

"I don't look too happy," I say.

"It's just your face," she says.

The box of crayons is turned such that I can see some of the label.

*24 Bold Colors*
*Encourages Self-Expression*
*Resistant to Bending and Breaking*

---

**JUSTIN MILLAN** is a writer and registered nurse working in New England.

ESSAY

# Things I Learned from Pole Dancing That I Did Not Learn from Residency

ELISE MULLAN

I WAS IN my second year of residency then. There was a lot going on. I was angry about COVID and tired of working nights. I missed sunlight. I felt stagnant. Despite all the hours I was putting in at the hospital, I didn't feel that I was becoming a better doctor. I drank more coffee. And then more lattes. In the interest of efficiency, I switched to shots of espresso. Something needed to change.

Rather than reflect on "What makes me happy?," in a fit of frustration I asked myself a different question: "What is the opposite of being a doctor?" And thus, I ended up in an "Intro to Pole Dancing" class.

The history of pole dancing is inextricably linked with sex and nightlife and more sex, and one could write a whole separate article on the misconceptions and stereotypes that led me to take that class. Mostly I wanted to do something that no one would expect me to do. Maybe I wanted to do something that people would not want me to do. For the first time in my life, at twenty-nine and three quarters, I felt angry enough to give in to the rebellious phase I skipped in high school (because when you only know how to do things the "proper" way, taking a new dance class feels bold).

In the first class, we learned two basic spins—a back hook spin and a dip turn. These are ground-level tricks, only requiring that you float inches off the floor. Still, I was hooked, and four months later I was in a level two class, hanging upside down from the ceiling. There was "the martini," where you sit in a pike position, so the combination of your body and pole resembles a tapered glass, and "the chopper," in which you throw your legs over your head like the fins on the top of a helicopter. I remember that on the Saturday before Easter I learned a new trick nicknamed "the crucifix," which I found particularly ironic.

In medicine, we draw strict boundaries around what is and what is not "professional." In the hospital, it's what you wear, how many piercings or tattoos you have, what you say, and how you conduct the exam. Despite the fact that marijuana is legal in many states, urine drug screens are common at the start of employment, and at federal health care facilities, any type of drug use is grounds for dismissal. So, in this environment, I wonder where pole dancing falls. What if it is a recreational activity? What if it is for exercise? And what if you do it for money? Can you still be a doctor?

The women and men who teach the pole dancing classes are athletes, coaches, and dancers. It takes an enormous amount of upper body and core strength to pull oneself up a stainless-steel pole, and the slower a trick is performed the less you can rely on momentum to get your body where it needs it to go. When it is done right it looks like ballet—effortless. There is basic physics to this art form as well. Words from my pre-med classes gained new relevance: "centrifugal force," "centripetal force," and "angular velocity." From practice you quickly learn that the smaller the radius, the faster you spin. And so, in letting go of the pole, in shooting your arms or legs out, the radius increases and you actually gain more control.

A pole, in comparison to a hospital, is laughingly simple. The hospital is composed of layers upon layers of administration, technology, insurance, complicated anatomy and physiology, and the individual needs of patients. It is impossible to see the whole hospital from any one vantage point. As a doctor, I have a grossly inadequate knowledge of insurance. Despite the fact that I regularly order numerous medications for patients, in the hospital it is the nurses and pharmacists who actually know what the medications look like. They are the ones who know exactly how they are given; which medications can be run through the same IV and which ones need separate access points.

There is not much to say about a pole. It should be straight, and sturdy enough to hold your weight. In Pictionary, you can draw it accurately without lifting your pen off the paper. Outside the hospital this simplicity felt like an exhale. I liked that when I climbed up the pole it was just me and the pole. It was what my body could do or not do. Both the accomplishments and the bruises were mine alone. There is a sense of fear when you climb to the top that reduces things to what matters most in that moment (getting down safely). You don't think about the complicated things like your to-do list (the laundry that is still unfolded next to the trash that really should be taken out), the half-finished applications for future jobs/fellowships/grants, and the nightly wondering about when your life is going to settle down so you can get pregnant and hoping that point intersects with a point when you are still fertile.

In stark contrast to the baggy scrubs worn on inpatient days or the slacks and dresses that compose the uniform of the outpatient clinic, most pole dancing students opt to wear sports bras and bathing suit bottoms. The higher you climb and the more complicated the tricks you attempt, the more excess clothing becomes an impediment. I would even argue that wearing more can make pole dancing dangerous because it is solely the friction of your skin on the pole that keeps you from falling all the way to the ground. So here, surface area matters. I had a strange revelation while struggling to sit five feet above the ground during one class. There was the briefest of moments in which I wished my thighs were larger. I swallowed the thought immediately.

Having grown up in a world signaling over and over again that the only option was for a woman's body to be smaller, the thought felt sacrilegious. Even now I cannot help but return to that moment, grateful and still puzzled by this shift in perspective. I discovered that there was an option between the two extremes for my body to be enough as it is, and in this thought there was relief.

During my first Intro to Pole class the teacher told us we could record ourselves and what we had learned at the end of the class. I didn't do it. I didn't want to see my body in a crop top and shorts. I cringed at the thought of there being video evidence of me stiffly attempting a seductive walk around the pole. But by the second class I was convinced to try it, and at the third class I willingly pulled out my phone at the end. The result is that I have accumulated a library of thirty-second clips just for me. They are little reminders of how I have grown and what I have learned, which I lean on when residency is hard.

Over the past year there have been moments when I felt so exhausted and unmotivated that I wondered if I had made a mistake in pursuing a career as a doctor. Learning to climb a pole was a sprinkle of glitter in the darkness. It was a little giggle. It was something a little unexpected and something new. When I started taking classes in February, it was a buoy that gave me something to look forward to each week. This was how I made it through March, then April, then on to July. I kept climbing the pole and enjoying the slide back down. I think in medicine and in life, we frequently get stuck in a tangle of expectations about who we should be and what we should do. Here, eight feet above ground, I found an argument for giving myself an escape.

---

**ELISE MULLAN** is a neurologist practicing in Massachusetts. Her work has been published in *Globe*, *Student Doctor Network*, and *Neurology*. She is a recipient of the American Academy of Neurology's 2025 Resident and Fellow Section Writing Award. "Things I Learned from Pole Dancing That I Did Not Learn from Residency" was recognized as a notable essay in the 2023 edition of *The Best American Essays*.

ESSAY

# Coming Out of the Medical Closet

ANGELICA RECIERDO

IT'S THE KIND of chill that is felt only in meat lockers and hospital stock rooms. I was in the latter, amid plastic-wrapped tools that only rubber-gloved hands are certified to touch.

She was a couple of inches adjacent to me, searching for a nasal cannula. The distance between us was approximately the length that the wrist is distal to the elbow. Her brow was furrowed and I could see the night shift seeping into her eyes. Her breath warmed the room a bit, giving some vitality to the otherwise menacing display of gleaming tubes and metal surfaces.

I looked at her and hoped to transmit the most empathy I could muster at 3 AM. I gave her a look of solidarity because no one else could ever understand what this feels like. I'm sure much heartache takes place within the walls of a medical closet. But I can attest that that is where courage is found again. We are nurses.

It took me a while to become comfortable just entering a patient's room. How could my feeble presence ever put someone at ease? I gulped in intimidation when seeing life-sustaining machines connected to every possible orifice and wires tangling my path to them like an obstacle course. I cringed when asking, "How are you doing?" resulted in a painful grunt or a labored "Oh, fine."

As a novice, you find yourself at a loss for words around people who are sick or in pain. You feel helpless, so you do the physiological tasks and scurry off. Then you progress and you stand a bit taller, wearing your stethoscope like a medallion around your neck. You garner some small-talk skills and warm up to simple starters like "Where's home for you?" or "Oh yeah, *Family Feud* is a riot."

Then one day, you surprise yourself. You'll be sitting with your ventilated patient and the silence will be comforting. The whir of their breathing apparatus will be soothing. You'll talk to them with ease, as if there's a cup of coffee between you.

As far as communication goes, the five senses become your greatest tools of operation. They will be sharpened under many cases and the fine-tuned detective within you will emerge.

It's a wonder how a murmur isn't a low whisper exchanged in conversation, that the whites of your eyes could be yellow or blue or that there's nothing scarier than a lump that won't go away. You become a storyteller of the body. You appreciate its honesty—symptoms arising for a reason, most likely because of some imbalance.

You become frustrated at those committing the typical health care sins, like smoking, or eating fatty foods. And you'll also be frustrated at those who had nothing to do with their prognosis other than being born. Karma and fate will try to explain themselves, but let compassion crush them both.

Birth and death are daily companions, the transitions of both always accompanied by a held breath. You'll hold your breath waiting for that initial cry from a newborn, muscles relaxing because you know that's the first sign of life—a triumphant, vocal declaration of survival. And you'll hold your breath once more as your dying patient slips away under layers of morphine.

My mind would always drift to "firsts" and "lasts" during these occasions. When is the first time this baby will laugh? Who did this dying man last say "I love you" to? You find yourself filling in the gaps of stories lost.

There are probably few places where humanity more genuinely surfaces than in a hospital: mothers gripping children's hands tighter before life-changing appointments, husbands leaning over stretchers, stealing one last kiss before surgery. I can't think of a more wretched place to be than in waiting, your mind riddled with everything that could go wrong.

These people are static, inhabiting waiting room chairs heavily—momentarily on pause. Humans shouldn't go through this alone. You remember your role, offering them a glass of water, and they look up at you, eyes pricked with tears. They sigh longer than anyone else. Their shoulders collapse, and you instill in them the same courage you found for yourself in the medical closet.

---

**ANGELICA RECIERDO** is a poetry editor for *Intima*, the author of the chapbook *One Last Ripe Life*, and a journalism and health impact fellow at the University of Toronto. She earned an MS in narrative medicine from Columbia University, a BS in nursing from Northeastern University, and an MFA in creative writing from Dominican University of California.

POEM

# Becoming a Doctor

BRENT SCHNIPKE

I've split the head of a donated man,
teased out his eyeballs, probed his skull,
carved his lungs, scrutinized his heart,
held his disembodied bones and bifurcated
brain. I've forgotten his name.

I've committed acts which other contexts
would render criminal.
I've counted gallstones, counted bruises,
slid needles between knuckles, sucked out
yellow human fluid. I've asked questions of others
I would never ask myself.

I've sewn fiber lines into veins,
thrust plastic tubes down throats.
I've smelled blood and bile,
bone glue and burning flesh.
I've seen knees sawed, spines screwed,

babies born, chests cracked, toes in jars,
death.

I've stitched skin
and split wounds open,
disemboweled babies
in the name of healing.
I've born witness
to the ugly and the holy,
and at times been the vessel
for both. I've listened to a dying woman
name her joys and fears, dying
not among them. I've wept.

I've handed a woman
her firstborn child.
I've saved lives by listening,
I've hurt by failing
to pay close enough attention.

I've been mistaken as the doctor,
and I've finally started to see it myself.
I've prayed with people on the brink
of the unknown, cringed
at my ineptitude, laughed
at the absurdity of it all. I've attended

to the gruesome and the divine,
in the name of learning
to be your doctor.

---

**BRENT SCHNIPKE** is an instructor in psychiatry and behavioral sciences and an attending psychiatrist in consultation-liaison psychiatry at Northwestern University.

ESSAY

# Getting to Know Dying

ANNA BELC

AFTER TWO YEARS of working as a labor and delivery nurse, I knew how to recognize imminent birth. The vomiting and shakes at seven centimeters dilation. The "I can't do it" and "Make it stop" at nine centimeters. The deep groans of pushing. I saw head after head emerge. I knew the signs. I knew when to keep the physician at bedside. When to keep gloves on.

And now, a year into working in the emergency room, I'm starting to learn the signs of imminent death. Five years as a nurse, yet the first time I saw it death took me by surprise. A patient came in sick, and I expected the blood cultures, the fluids, the antibiotics, a transfer to the intensive care unit. I didn't expect the sudden pain and pallor, the absent pulse. Then the call to the operator for help, the crash cart, hands on chest, shock pads, epinephrine, sodium bicarb, etc. etc. etc.

It happens again and again and again.

The daughter of an eighty-seven-year-old just-deceased mother says, "But how can I leave her?" She stands a foot away from the stretcher, her hand trembling, almost reaching. Earlier, before she arrived, I struggled to remove her mother's wedding ring from her finger. I knew I would have to be rough and didn't want her to watch. I washed her hair, tried the lube and the shampoo cap to remove the blood, then resolved to bandage the wound. "Thank you for taking care of her," the daughter says, and I wonder whether she means while dead or while alive. I walk her father, the husband, to the bathroom. He holds steady. I wonder if, at their age, he expected it. "My ninety-year-old legs don't work that well anymore," he says as I walk slowly next to him. He's putting one foot in front of another with no walker, no cane. "I only hope at ninety my legs work this well," I tell him.

I still can't remember on which ankle and which wrist the death tags go. But I know how to tie them now. That night on my way out of the hospital, my own boots poorly tied, my jacket unzipped, I see the transporter walk with a covered gurney and I open the morgue door for him. I'm out the door into sunlight for once, because she died at 6:47 AM and I didn't leave until 8, the sun finally up above Lake Superior, my boots crunching on fresh snow, thinking again how beautiful this place is, and how remote.

In the process of getting to know death I start to wonder how those who walk through our ER doors might die. I do not want to be taken by surprise. In nursing school, I was taught to anticipate the worst in order to take the best care of our patients. I need to think of the exact mechanism of their death so that I am best prepared to prevent it.

A man with a gastrointestinal bleed will, of course, bleed to death. Someone with an infection will die of septic shock. A post-surgical patient will develop a pulmonary embolism. So I insert large-bore IVs in both arms' antecubitals for a rapid blood transfusion. I study blood pressure trends in case I need to give fluids before the patient becomes dangerously hypotensive. I leave bruise after bruise injecting blood thinners.

Still, there is that moment when in the middle of dancing around each other hooking up the cardiac monitor, taking a manual blood pressure, confirming verbal orders, cursing under my breath that a piece of equipment is missing, I stop and realize: This person is dying. A moment of reverence for the knowledge the patient and I hold alone. I know it is coming because the dying know it is coming. They fight for each breath, fighting us to sit straight up, to get up, to do something other than die, right there on our hand-cranked stretcher. Family unaware; panicked but relieved to have nurses and doctors crowding the room, working. I want the family to read my mind, but I don't want them to meet my eye. I now know birth and death intimately. I have also seen the intersection of the two. To make it easier on ourselves we called them IUFDs, which, looking back, sounds like extraterrestrial sightings instead of the real tragedies of an obstetric unit.

Intrauterine fetal demises.

I have seen infants born still. And I have seen them be born and die. The stethoscope used to listen for their heartbeat larger than their chest. Eyes barely able to open. Webbing between fingers. Their toes their only perfection. We were taught at obstetric orientation that if families want photos and you can't bear to take a photo of the entirety of the infant then take photos of feet. Feet are always perfect, no matter how early. I've spent too long in a cold, brightly lit operating room, where they say the lighting is best, behind the camera, arranging letter blocks to spell out the child's name or the word "Angel." Then, after, later, the death tag wrapped around the whole body. Where that tag goes is easy to remember.

So many tips on how to prepare the dead yet none on how to prepare the living. During orientation, no one prepared me for the moment the paramedics call on their radio and ask for the physician, something they only do when they need one to declare a time of death. No one warned me a woman would tell me she feels legs in her vagina, her tiny breech infant being born weeks before he is ready to survive. So, I take too long arranging their feet and hands. I take too long with the ritual, getting to know death, the dying, the dead.

---

**ANNA BELC** is a NICU nurse in Minneapolis and a mother of four. She was born and raised in Poland, attended school in New York

City, and as an adult fell in love with Philadelphia, where she studied theater and, later, nursing. Her most impactful work was in a rural ER in Michigan's Upper Peninsula on the shores of Lake Superior. For her, home is wherever it snows.

SHORT STORY

# Night Watch

DANA GAGE

RANE ENTERED THE room hesitantly; she didn't want to enter at all. She had pleaded with the intern and then the resident, who just shook his head and said it wasn't up to him: the chief resident had ordered—had insisted upon it—that she see this particular child, work her up. Her protests had ended with a plea for mercy on the child's behalf, earning her another demerit in the chief resident's assessment of her performance: refusing an assignment. His list of complaints about her was long. She could recite them all: failure to work up an admission (even though she had done seven that night), failure to write her notes promptly (even though she was in class until 3 PM every day), and finally, failure to attend grand rounds (when she had taken a child to CT scan because everyone else was busy).

In the darkened room, Rane looked at the woman huddling in the shadows, then at the little girl on the bed. She appeared to be about six. Her hair was gone, and on her scalp, nodules protruded from the bony surface. Her eyes were half open, glazed. Her arms and legs were also covered with nodules, bony, stretching the skin tight. The flesh around them seemed to have evaporated, as if all nourishment had given over to feeding them, leaving the girl with nothing. The rest of her skin was pale and pressed shiny and smooth over her abdomen, filled with fluid, a ball of fluid pinning her to the bed. Her umbilicus pushed outward as if she were ready to give birth. With each shallow breath came a little moan, as if that small effort was more than she could bear. In the reflected light, Rane stared into the face of death.

What Rane saw left her wondering how she could touch this child, what she could do, how she could justify such an invasion.

Outside the door she saw the chief resident approach; he stood watching, waiting, wanting to make sure his instructions were carried out.

She turned to the mother. "Why are you still here? It's late. Don't you want to go home and get some rest? Your other children, I saw them before."

The woman nodded and Rane followed her gaze; two toddlers lay tangled together on a cot in the corner.

"Shouldn't they be home?" she asked. "Your husband . . ."

"They want to be here. With their sister; they miss her at home." She spoke firmly. "My husband? I haven't seen him in weeks. We take turns. When he's not working one of his three jobs to pay for this care she is receiving. The best. We wanted the best, the number one doctor in this area. Ha! What did it matter? And now. Another round of chemo they say, just give it a chance; it might buy her some time, time to go home." The woman bent over to muffle a sob.

She looked at Rane again.

"Just let us go home," she pleaded. "Why won't they just let us go home? Why can't she die in her own bed?"

"You still have hope," Rane said. "There's always that."

The woman looked up suddenly and stared at Rane. "I know who you are; they told me about you, that you would be in here to see my daughter. You're pretty special, I hear, doing your own bone research, already getting ready to publish a paper, only a freshman but cutting a notch for yourself. Number One, another Number One."

"We all want to be the best at something," said Rane.

"And what do you have to offer my daughter? What new

treatment plan? What new drug?"

The only light in the child's room was reflected from a spotlight on the corner of the building. It shone mostly on the parking lot, the cars huddling like bears waiting for prey. Rane moved forward, and as she approached the bed, there was stirring.

"Can't you leave her alone?" the woman said.

"Ma'am?"

"What is it with you people? She's just barely fallen asleep. What do you want with my daughter?

Rane stopped.

"Please don't touch the bed. It hurts her so bad. Could she get more pain meds?"

"I'll talk to them for you; just let me do this first. I have to do a physical exam, take a history."

"When you touch her, she screams in pain. Surely you can get her something. She's dying. Isn't that enough? Can't you see that?"

"I'm not sure what they have planned."

"So they sent you in here to learn from my daughter, who can't bear to have someone breathe on her? They told you to come and examine her?"

Rane stopped and took a deep breath. "Yes, ma'am. But I told them I wouldn't do it. And they told me my career is on the line."

The woman got up from the chair and took a washcloth from the bedside table, dipped it in a kidney basin of water. Rane watched as the woman struggled to bend over her daughter and keep her balance. She took the cloth and held it just over her daughter's forehead, not touching but close enough to diffuse the coolness onto her daughter's flushed face, soothing by intention only. No direct contact.

Then she looked over at Rane. "Do you know what it is like to lose something so precious to you? Do you? Do you know what it is like not to be able to comfort your dying daughter in your arms?" She paused. "Isn't there anything you can give her?"

"The medicine is so strong; they are afraid to give her more. It will slow her breathing, cause her to . . ."

"What? Die?" The woman began to laugh in a high-pitched keen, rocking back and forth on her heels, then breaking into great raw sobs. When Rane reached out to her, she snapped back just out of reach.

"That's the medical stance, isn't it? Can't give the dying patient too much pain medication or it might kill them. Better to let them feel every moment of suffering along the way, let them suffer their death as long as they can. Tell me why it is necessary for this little girl to feel every moment of pain? Tell me. For what?" Again, she started to sob, but cut herself short when the tangle of her other children started to stir.

"Well, I can tell you one thing, Miss Number One in the Class. You are not going to touch my daughter; I don't care if you flunk out of school. You will not lay one hand on her. Do you understand?"

In the dark room, Rane's eyes had adjusted to the light. She could see the woman's face.

"You're right, ma'am. I won't touch her. Now just sit down and try to rest. I will sit here with her until morning. Let me just check this IV rate and I'll make sure her pain meds are running smoothly. You sit. I'll be with her. And I swear to you that I will not touch her. Would you mind if I said a few prayers that my grandmother taught me? It might soothe her."

---

**DANA GAGE,** a founding editor of *Intima*, has been a practicing physician since 1978, concentrating on emergency, internal, forensic, and narrative medicine. She grew up in a small town in upstate New York, delivered by the same physician who cared for her entire family. Gage has spoken at numerous medical conferences. She is working on a novel about a medical student of Native American heritage, and a collection of stories based on her experiences as a prison doctor.

ESSAY

# Body of Work

ANNA DOVRE

The cadaver is so small that my first thought, glimpsing her frame through the thin white blanket, is that she's been dismembered from the chest down. All I can discern is the rounded skull, the hint of a nose, two knobs of shoulder.
 On the wall behind me, daylight seeps in through tall frosted windows. The conditioned air bounces off stainless steel cabinets and porcelain sinks. On the back of the door, a whiteboard proclaims in a large, curling script, "Be like a sponge: absorb knowledge!" We are third- and fourth-year medical students, here to practice emergency skills on a cadaver. I wear a loaner set of scrubs in mismatched shades of green, and the cloth is stiff against my goosebump-covered skin. I wonder who wore them last.
 For our first exercise, we will learn about airway management. The tools sit on a wheeled stand next to the cadaver table, various tubes and blades and syringes in orderly rows. Our instructor pulls down the blanket far enough to reveal a head wrapped in cloth and gauze, with only the mouth uncovered. Her jaw is slackened, her cheeks hollow, and her mouth—empty of teeth—gapes open in a perfect, shadowed O. I want to place my warm hands along those cheeks, to peel the bandages off her eyes, to cradle that tiny head in the crook of my arm. And I also want to run away.

The point here seems simple: corpse as proxy for one's own mortality. But looking at a cadaver doesn't remind me of death; rather, illness, decay, and the separation of the body into its constituent parts—skin, muscle, bone, fat. There's no mystery in a cadaver, because dissection is the procedural excision of mystery. A more apt metaphor for death would be something akin to a black hole, the event horizon, the point from which there is quite literally no return.

---

I stand at the head of the bed, preparing for intubation. Curved like a scythe, the dull metal instrument in my left hand catches the light. I place my right palm over the cadaver's covered forehead, press gently, and her head tilts back. There's debris in her mouth, on the back of her tongue, flecks of dried blood and something else, which coats the surface of my gloved thumb as I grasp her jaw and pull forward. Once I find her vocal cords—those pearly gates—the tube goes in easily. Next to me, a classmate squeezes on a firm plastic balloon, puffing artificial breaths into stiff lungs. I watch the rise and fall of her chest, a miraculous puppetry. Our instructor nods, once. The breaths cease, the tube is removed, and we rotate around the table to do it all again.

---

In my early twenties, I volunteered in a hospice program. Among the list of available duties— errands, clerical work, selling plush toys at the gift store—I chose to be a "companionship" volunteer. At the time, death held a comfortably abstract role in my life, a gritty concept to be mused over in basement apartments and sprinkled into essays on Samuel Beckett. I sought a first-hand, transcendental experience; only in retrospect do I see this for the privilege it was. After a few training sessions held in an office building on the outskirts of town, my phone number was added to a spreadsheet and I was deemed ready: a capable companion for the dying.

When the first call came, I drove to the nursing home with my stomach in knots. I had a name, a room number, and a folder full of pamphlets telling me what death ought to look like. The room was warm, sparsely decorated, the twin bed pushed up against the window. There was a bottle of lotion on the bedside table, and a Bible. I introduced myself to her, told her I'd stay awhile, though she appeared to be sleeping or comatose or otherwise—in some fundamental way, elsewhere. (Even as we lose our senses, the pamphlets say, hearing remains. How they know this I cannot say.) I rubbed lotion into the tissue-paper skin of her knuckles and counted her irregular, rasping breaths until my shift was over. She was "actively dying."

This is what I remember most from our hospice training class: that there are different ways to die. To die actively means the pauses between breaths lengthen and stutter; the mind slips into unconsciousness; the skin begins to mottle into starbursts of purple and blue. To die inactively—well, that becomes a question of semantics, of philosophy. Years later, a palliative care doctor would tell me, "There's a difference between living longer and dying slowly." As though that difference should be obvious.

---

We learn a lot from our cadaver: after intubation come chest tubes, intraosseous lines, surgical airways. The chest tube is the most technically challenging, leveraging a thick plastic tube up and over the rib into the lung space. By the time it's my turn, she already has several holes in her side, and so I follow the paths left behind. At some point, standing at the foot of the table, taking stock of all the places we've poked and sliced and drilled and sewn her, a snippet of song drifts into my mind: *Your body is a wonderland.* I wonder who to tell this to. And then I wonder at myself: the way my nausea has ebbed, my body looser, at ease. If anything, the scene on the table has become more gruesome, but perhaps that has rendered her less real, less human to me.

I witnessed my first death in a bustling emergency department on the edge of the Great Plains, where snowshoe hares would graze at the edge of the parking lot. It was my second week on the job; in the trauma bay, a man was strapped under a CPR machine that pumped his chest with a relentless metallic fervor. The sound this made was like the pressing in and out of a freshness seal on a bottle cap. One of his arms hung off the edge of the bed and shook in concert with the machinated compressions.

At some point there was a pause, a checking of the pulse, a decision made in a series of glances. Then the machine was unhooked, the IV lines removed, the blanket pulled up over the body. The hospital chaplain arrived: I remember her knitted white cardigan, worn over a canary yellow shirt with embroidered lapels. She recited a prayer with her palms spread open, as if to catch rain. At the end, she said, "May all in this room know that the place between life and death is a holy one."

We slipped one by one out of that holy room. Someone taped a paper image of a dove onto the doorframe, and we went on with our work. He went downstairs to the morgue. On the electronic patient list, his icon turned a maroon color, the word "expired" materializing in the comment section like an omen. I felt unchanged.

In medicine, the concept of "mortality" carries a specific, epidemiological meaning, often uttered alongside—and in conversation with—the concept of "morbidity." These terms live in symbiosis, affectionately referred to as M&M: Morbidity, the state of illness, and Mortality, its terminus. When I first heard of an "M&M conference," I was disappointed to learn its purpose: that of reviewing adverse patient outcomes, the unexpected accrual of death and disease. On close review, such misfortunes (a patient falling ill, experiencing an unexpected complication, or indeed dying) may in some cases belie an error in medical practice. The goal, then, is to identify the error and prevent it from happening again. Morbid as the human condition is, many of these cases are found to be unavoidable—a reminder that what's mortal is destined to be so.

---

When I return home from the cadaver lab, I shower and let the water run till it turns cold. Afterward, I stand in front of the mirror, the fluorescent light abuzz. Along the shadowed column of my neck, I trace the knobs of my trachea, find the thyroid and cricoid cartilages and the ribbon of membrane spanning them. I turn to the side and lift one arm, running my hand along the imaginary line from armpit to hip. We look so different, the cadaver and I. Perhaps I am trying to understand death through comparison. Her fat and muscle had melted away, her skin pulled taught across the scaffolding of her ribcage. On my own chest, subcutaneous tissue obscures the outlines of bone, so I have to find each rib by touch, feeling them lift into my palm with every breath. I pause below my fifth rib, testing the skin, trying to work my finger into the space between the bones. I picture a scalpel making that first incision: dark blood welling in its wake, the pop of punctured pleura, a length of tube sliding in deep, snaking up through my chest, and at last coming to rest in a dark, soft corner, close to my heart.

---

There's a planetarium half a mile from my home, where a man named Thaddeus holds court among the stars. On a cold day in early December, two months after the cadaver lab, I walk to the planetarium along streets bleached bone white with salt. About a dozen of us claim seats under the darkened dome, necks tilted back against cushioned headrests, as Thaddeus takes us five billion years into the future: the day when the Milky Way galaxy will collide with our nearest neighbor, Andromeda. He shows us the collision, slowed down and projected onto the concave screen: two swirls of sparkling dust, catching one another's outstretched arms like partners in a dance. In the heat and gravitational pressure of their joining, Thaddeus says, new stars will be born. "Maybe we'll be able to move to one of them," he says.

 I admire his intergalactic optimism, his belief in a collective immortality spanning eons, light-years of humanity stretched over an impossible horizon. I do not agree with Thaddeus. The finitude of my existence, and of our species, is one of the few things of which I am certain. Here is the scale, I think, at which death is its most comforting: a glorious doomsday of staggering scope, so far in the distance that it might as well be fiction. I imagine a dust-strewn dawn, the scattered and flighty particles of my long-dead body caught in orbital eddies, burning and gold-limned by the light of a thousand new stars. And it doesn't scare me at all.

---

**ANNA DOVRE** is a family medicine resident in Saint Paul, Minnesota, where she lives with her wife and dog. She enjoys fantasy novels, baked goods, and stinky cheeses. Her work has been published in *The Examined Life Journal* and *Family Medicine*.

# 2

# A THIN LINE

*Love and Hate*

SHORT STORY

# Pretending Not to Know

PRISCILLA MAINARDI

DORITOS FOR BREAKFAST, at 7 AM. I scoop up a handful from the open bag on the desk at the nurses' station. They're chewy, as if they've been sitting there for days. Kat, the night nurse, tells me about a new patient. "Rosalie Romero, forty-nine, came in with infected hardware in her right femur. Dr. Harvey removed it yesterday in the OR and put in a new rod and screws. There's a dressing on her thigh but you can't see much of it because her leg is in a brace. She has MS and needs a lot of help. Can you take her some Tylenol? She has a headache. I just got the order."

We have to call a doctor for every order, even Tylenol. Kat glances around the nurses' station to see who's nearby, then drops her voice. "This is the woman who murdered her husband, out in Chester County."

I stop writing and look up from Rosalie's printout. This is more than I need to know.

I'm wary enough with new patients, not knowing what to expect, and this adds another dimension. I'd rather think of her as an ordinary suburban housewife, whose physical troubles I can deal with and whose emotional ones are largely left at home. But murdering your husband is too big to leave at home and will have to be dealt with somehow, by both of us, so I can take care of her.

"Who knows about this?" I say to Kat.

"Everyone. It happened a couple of months ago. She shot him

in the back, from her wheelchair. Her kids were asleep down the hall."

One more thing I don't want to know, that I can't unknow. "Don't worry," Kat says. "I've got your back."

"Oh, don't. Please," I say, biting my lip to keep from laughing. Because what's funny, really, about a woman with MS who's accused of murder?

I walk down the hall to Rosalie's room, reminding myself of the effects of multiple sclerosis on the brain and nervous system: decreased attention span, poor judgment, memory loss, difficulty reasoning and solving problems. Suppose pulling the trigger was just another symptom of the disease? I know both too much and too little about Rosalie, too much from what Kat told me, and too little, the way we can never really know another person. Here's what Rosalie doesn't know about me: that my thirteen-year-old daughter Belinda has been demanding to meet her father and isn't speaking to me because I can't find a way to tell her she's the result of a one-night stand with a drug felon.

Rosalie's room is dark. I go to the window and turn the blinds, letting in little slivers of light.

"Hello, my name is Devon," I say, the way I always do. "I'll be your nurse today."

Her long dark hair is tangled all over the pillow. She opens her eyes. One eye looks at me while the other strays to the window. "Did you bring the Tylenol?"

"Yes. Tell me about the pain." I set the cup with her morning medications on her overbed table and pour her some water.

"My leg's okay," she says, "it's just my head."

"Can you give me a number?" I point to the zero to ten pain scale tacked to the wall by the bed. I need the number for my notes. I also need description, pattern, duration, when it started, where it radiates, what helps it, and what makes it worse, but I don't bother with these right now.

"Eleven," she says. She lifts her arm so I can scan her name-band, then dumps the pills onto the table. She picks out the two Tylenols, puts them in her mouth, and swallows them dry.

"Leave the others," she says. "I'll take them later."

We're not supposed to leave pills lying around but I don't argue. I put them back in the cup and leave it on the table. "I need to look you over," I say.

Rosalie closes her eyes and turns on her side. "I'm fine. Can't you just get out?"

I want to, but I have a sudden vision of her leg, the dressing saturated, blood pooling on the sheet and dripping down the side of the bed to form a sticky puddle on the floor. I lift the blankets and take a quick peek. She's right. She's fine.

I escape then, relieved to return to the warmth and activity of the nurses' station. But the lights in the hallway seem too bright, giving off a toxic fluorescent hum. I stand for a moment at the med cart. That wasn't the scrupulously good care I'd planned to give Rosalie, to prove to myself that I wasn't blaming or judging her.

"What's the story?" I say to Dr. Harvey at ten thirty. He's sitting at the desk with her chart. "Why is she here? Why not in jail?"

"She made bail, and she needed the surgery." He shrugs, as if he operates on patients who are out on bail every day. "How is she?"

"She won't do anything. She threw me out. Threw Becky out, threw out physical therapy."

"She's depressed, but she won't hurt anyone," Dr. Harvey says. "She needs to get up and moving, do her therapy, especially with the MS. At least get her sitting on the side of the bed. She's wheelchair bound anyway." He stands, shaking his head. "What a bum deal. I'll go talk to her."

"Please," I say.

Dr. Harvey comes back a few minutes later. "I laid down the law," he says, writing an order in the chart. "She'll cooperate. Can you change her dressing, Devon?" He hands me the chart.

"Why'd she shoot him?" I say.

"Allegedly," he says. "She allegedly shot him. They were in the middle of a divorce. They were arguing."

He makes it all sound so plausible, reasonable even. I wonder why she frightens me. She can't hurt me, and our situations aren't even similar. I don't have MS or a gun, or even a husband.

I go back to her room when the lunch trays come. Rosalie has turned on the light and is eating dry Cheerios, with the phone pressed to her ear. She gives me a brief smile, one of those down-turned ones where the lips barely move. While I wait for her to hang up, I straighten her belongings: an open package of chocolate chip cookies, her hairbrush and makeup case.

"In my dream," she says into the phone, "I was walking and my legs worked fine." There's a pause, then she says, "I gotta go. The nurse is here. I had such a terrible headache this morning I think I scared this poor nurse." She hangs up and gives me the almost smile again.

I smile, accepting her indirect apology. "Headache better?"

"Much."

"Okay if I change your dressing now?"

She nods. I lift the covers. Dr. Harvey left the Velcro straps of the brace undone, and the old dressing, brown with dried blood, dangles from her thigh. I remove it and toss it in the trash, then tape fresh gauze over her incision, which is closed with clips that look like short, fat staples.

I refasten the brace and wash my hands in the bathroom, looking at myself in the mirror above the sink. I look the same as I did yesterday, and the day before, and the day before that, though in theory I'm a different person today than I was yesterday and I'll be another person tomorrow. Who can say I won't someday be a person who has murdered my husband, who will need surgery due to complications from MS, who will need a nurse to help me and will need that nurse to pretend she doesn't know the first thing about me?

Rosalie's phone is ringing again when I come out of the bathroom. She ignores it. "Probably my mother," she says. "I don't feel like talking to her right now. I told her I was lonely and you know what she said? I shouldn't have shot my husband if I didn't want to be alone."

"That must be difficult," I say, drawing on a stock nursing phrase.

"It was a joke, Devon," she says. "You can smile."

So I do. "Do you want to talk about it?" I say. Pretending not to know isn't helping anyone.

"It's all such a mess," Rosalie says, shaking her head. She raises herself on her elbows. "I'd like to get in the wheelchair for lunch if you'll help me."

I lift her shoulders and pull her around until her legs dangle off the side of the bed. She combs out her tangled hair while I unfold the wheelchair, pressing down on the seat with both hands. I help slide her into the chair and move the overbed table in front of her, glad to return to the realm of the physical; perhaps this is, after all, the best way I can help her.

I bundle her dirty linen into a ball. I smooth clean white sheets on the bed and turn them down so the bed is ready for her when she wants to get back in.

That night at home I turn down my own sheets, but I don't get in bed. I go down the hall to Belinda's room to tell her about her father.

---

**PRISCILLA MAINARDI** is a writer and editor living in New Jersey. Her short stories and essays, many of them inspired by her work as a registered nurse at a community hospital, have appeared in *Pulse*, *The Examined Life Journal*, the literary magazine *bioStories*, and *Atticus Review*. She earned her MFA in creative writing from Rutgers University - Newark, where she taught English composition. Mainardi is a fiction editor for *Intima*.

ESSAY

# Love, Frank

## CHERYL BAILEY

"Dr. Bailey, there's a basket here for you and Phyllis!" The receptionist from my oncology office heaves the delivery box onto the counter. Fruit skewers mimic a floral display with balls of cantaloupe, pineapple-chunk daisies, and strawberry roses. Clinic staff can't resist surrounding the bounty.

"Clever," I say, crinkling the cellophane as I retrieve the envelope. I'm nonchalant, but treats from a happy patient brighten the day and grant us all a breather from the chaos of office hours. Nothing cheers up an oncologist like food, though getting thanked in an obituary runs a close second.

"Who sent the arrangement?" asks my nurse Phyllis. She manages to appear uninterested but was the first to escape our corner cubicle for a look when she heard her name. I grin when I read the salutation and hand her the note. She chuckles.

"I can't believe it's been ten years. Good for her." She smiles, takes a fruit skewer, and heads back to work. Ever irritable, Phyllis pokes, "Room two's been ready for you for ten minutes. She's in a gown, and double-parked.

Time flies for women with ovarian cancer. The moment they hear the diagnosis, they also learn they have few days left to savor the world. It takes courage to dive into life knowing the cancer will recur, that at some point the chemo will stop working. Other gynecologic oncologists describe it as a chronic disease. I've never liked that analogy; ovarian cancer isn't high blood pressure.

But the patient who'd sent the fruit basket had dodged the miserable statistics. She was celebrating a mighty marker of survival—a decade since her initial diagnosis and surgery. After the radical pelvic surgery, she'd sailed through six cycles of chemotherapy. During clinic visits she regaled me with stories of working out while bald or flirting without eyebrows.

"You know how men at the gym check you out from the corners of their eyes? It used to be to see how much I was lifting. Now I think they want to figure out why I don't have hair. I'm ordering a t-shirt that says: TEMPORARY BALDNESS DURING CHEMO. HAIR BACK SOON, so they can relax around me." She worked full time, took care of other people's plants and animals, and stayed thoroughly, cheerfully engaged in the world.

"Would I be this fun on chemo?" I'd asked Phyllis after one of her follow-up visits. She sighed, with a hint of an eye roll. "You always see yourself in the young ones. Who knows how you'd react? Now, I'd love you to call Radiology while I room the next patient."

Phyllis nudged me along, making it clear, as always, that emotional matters were of no interest to her.

At another visit, the patient informed me, "People give me free stuff, you know. The bakery lady at Cub threw in a couple of extra bagels when she saw my bald head under the cap. And there's a guy at work who always brings me a piece of carrot cake the last week of the month. His wife makes it especially for me," she chattered through her pelvic exam, sitting up in the stirrups to punctuate a critical part of the tale. "I don't have the heart to tell him I hate carrot cake."

―

Months passed. One day she came to my office with bloating and abdominal pressure. She had a huge cystic mass in her pelvis, a slight increase in her tumor marker, and unrelenting pain. I took her back to the operating room, expecting it to be a last-ditch effort for a massive recurrence. Instead, everything looked great once I got the mass out.

Only problem? I couldn't spare her distal sigmoid. She woke up with a colostomy.

This is always tough news, but her coping style wasn't having it. She engaged with her stoma nurses and dove into learning about the colostomy appliances. ("They frown on the word 'bag,' Dr. Bailey, so I humor them," she'd told me). Weeks later she marched into my office, declaring, "Frank and I are doing just fine!"

I was caught off guard—had I forgotten she was in a new relationship? Was Frank her cat? She saw my confusion and explained, "My stoma. I named him Frank, the forward-facing a\*\*hole!" She and Frank thrived, with years of cancer-free health to follow.

Patients can be memorable for all sorts of personalities—some quirky, some terrible.

This insanely wonderful woman had always been a joy in the office, chatting up the receptionist, thanking the phlebotomist by name. She was independent, feisty, and optimistic. I liked to think I share those qualities, but hers were battle tested. I felt a little guilty as I tried to be a "cool" character in her cancer care. Phyllis, always accurate with getting back to patients, was especially quick to report tumor marker results to this woman before the ink was dry. The fact she could make Phyllis laugh over the phone? Miraculous.

At a visit a few years later, she leaned over to confide in the latest events in her life since the last checkup. "Well, I've had a little issue. I went out to that club on Highway 10, used to be called The Sea Cap'n. Cheap booze and country bands on Saturdays?" She raised her eyebrows, nodding at my grin.

I'd gone there with non-doctor friends during med school to smoke and drink, unseen by my classmates. "The wings," I sighed. "The wings were tremendous."

She nodded. "Yep, that's the one. Appetizers are still their thing. Anyhoo. The place changed owners, so my workmate and I went to check it out a few months ago and had a blast. Thing is, though, I just could not stop chewing on ice. Even made the waitress bring me a pitcher of it to chomp on while the band took a break."

The patient continued, "Well, as we were walking up to the dance floor, I grabbed a drained cocktail glass from an empty table and threw it back." She looked at me, daring me to comment.

"Wait. You drank out of a stranger's glass?"

She cackled. "Can you even believe that? Luckily my friend grabbed my arm when I reached for the second one and said, 'What the hell? Don't do that—you'll catch a disease!' Her disgusted expression snapped me back to reality, and I knew something was wrong. I'd been kind of obsessively chewing for a few weeks. Had to have something hard in my mouth to crack and chomp on."

"I went to my primary," she continued, hands waving in punctuation, "she checked some labs, and said I was vitamin deficient and anemic. Ever heard of pica, Doc?" she asked. "It's named after magpies, who evidently peck away at practically anything, food or not.

"That's what I had. She ordered an upper and lower GI—gah, Frank *loved* that whole scene—but there was no bleeding. It's always something, right?" She leaned back in her clinic chair, arms crossed to keep the cloth gown closed.

Pica is the condition in which people compulsively chew things, often dirt or clay. I recalled from residency the rare pregnant woman who would present with pica and have all sorts of labs and studies to make a treatment plan. The urge to chew usually went away after delivery.

"How are your teeth?" I asked. "Sometimes people crack them."

Her eyes gleamed as she squinted her way into a smile. "Just had a six-month cleaning, and they seem good. I'm pretty sure my dentist thinks I've got a mental disorder. There's a delicate balance between taking an iron supplement and keeping Frank happy, but the urge to chew is a lot less. Yep, Frank hates iron pills."

She reached into her purse to check her medical calendar. "Had my mammo last week, by the way. The girls are fine." She gazed at me over the cheaters she always kept hanging off a bright fabric lanyard.

"So it's just the tumor marker left. Do you have good news for me or am I gonna have to bite off a piece of your desk?"

I laughed, moving my hands to guard the edge. "No, no, keep taking your iron and leave my furniture alone! Your CA-125 is eight. Even lower than six months ago. That plus the normal CT scan a few months ago? You're in the clear."

The briefest of swallows from her clued me in. Her sass projected strength, but the possibility of recurrence was always on her mind. She stood, hopped on the exam table, and whooped, "Let's get on with it, then, doc. Frank and I've got places to go today. I've gotta tell everyone I'm good for another six months!"

I stood too. We were the same height. Same age. Strong personalities. Professional women. She was, I realized, *my* role model. If I ever needed chemo, I hoped my name on the day's clinic list would make someone smile.

Seeing her name did more than that for me. For one, the rare survivors reassure me I must have *some* skill, a *little* expertise, to have guided them through the minefields of ovarian cancer. As much as we oncologists might deny it, we stuff down the fear that our patients' deaths are our fault, that we're not good enough doctors to cure them. The survivors soothe our egos and keep us in the game. How ridiculous I was to feel proud that she, sparkling and alive, was my patient.

She also helped me confront my own fear of death. I identified with her, and as I watched this woman beating the odds, I was grateful to have lived those same years in health. Her very survival reminded me to appreciate my good fortune. Oncology magnifies that lesson every day.

As time passed, I grudgingly lengthened the interval between visits from six to twelve months. The risk of another recurrence was so small that the random visits were more for our comfort than any medical logic. She worked for some cranky lawyers, and I enjoyed hearing the stories about them, or about the neighbors who'd watched out for her after surgery and chemo. These characters became part of her clinic visits. Even Phyllis asked for an update if she missed the latest anecdote, still affecting her air of not *really* caring.

That day, the clinic staff resumed their frazzled work after taking some fruit. I brought the note back to my cubby, where Phyllis sat staring at the computer screen. Her skewer untouched, she was dabbing her eyes with a tissue. I read the note again.

*Dear Dr. Bailey and Phyllis,*

*Many thanks for the wonderful gift of ten years of life.*

*Love, Frank*

---

**CHERYL BAILEY** is a retired gynecologic oncologist who reviews articles for the *Journal of Medical Regulation*. She is the author of the novel *Poised*, which follows a Dr. Shelly Riley during her surgical training in 1990s Kentucky. Bailey lives in Saint Paul, Minnesota, with her husband, her mom, and two poorly behaved dogs.

ESSAY

# Yours

### NINA GABY

You carry the boxes out of your office while it's still light. A generic office in a general psychiatric clinic where you have spent moments of such sheer immersion that often you blink hard into the sunset at end of day, unsure and breathless.

Rifling through the papers, you realize these are papers from your last office. Actually, the one before that, which was the same facility you are now leaving again. No, the dates indicate another decade, another state. You wonder why you aren't able to stay in one place for more than a year and a half, sometimes less, convinced it's your fault but then realize no, it's the system and nothing is really going to improve no matter where you are. It's health care, after all.

The antique lamps that you think might be your mother's but maybe you are wrong about that—she's been gone so long now—are already packed in the car, supported by the oriental rug that you also drag from place to place. The rug and the lamps spiff up the office spaces you are assigned, especially if you don't get the windows you were promised. There's a particular peachy salmon that you generally paint your walls, a color that picks up shades of the border in the rug. The color goes back thirty years, to your first office. A rich and lucky color, like a gemstone, maybe like hope. This time you weren't allowed to paint the walls, and you didn't argue, as if it was very clear you wouldn't be staying. And this time you didn't hang the four large gesture drawings you did in an art residency a decade ago, before circumstances forced you to go back to work in the health care systems you thought you had escaped. What a relief not to have to carefully pack them today and feel bad about the holes you leave in the walls.

The next day you are unloading the car, having brought home the boxes full of papers, too lazy and dispirited to go through them in the office. Most of them should have gone to the shredder.

You start throwing papers into the woodstove. You make a separate pile with cards and notes from patients, from students, proof of worthiness and connection. Your hand hovers between that pile and the fire. In the other room there are boxes from another move. You toss the cards into one of those boxes and shut the woodstove. You left all this stuff around instead of hiding it in the barn, out of sight, out of mind. What's wrong with you? Once you left a box under the piano for over a year, unsure of how to let it go.

Wiping your hands on your sweatshirt, you go over and stand in front of the open refrigerator for a moment but nothing appeals so you go back to your task.

From the bottom of the farthest box you yank a manila envelope with an address from a police station in a distant state. The envelope looks old, the scuffed label handwritten, and you wonder how it got in the box from this office. You separate the frayed edges. Inside is a police report. Then you remember.

The patient was referred by their workplace for an evaluation after getting drunk and threatening a coworker. We will call the patient Sal. We will not identify a race, a gender, or an age. We can use the singular "they." We will just say that the contents of the envelope are almost an inch thick and include photographs. All this would now be digitized, its physicality shredded in that distant office in a distant state.

You will now recall the night you received it, several offices ago. Sal had come in for a few appointments, and after establishing you as a safe person (more invested in Sal than in Sal's employer) Sal told you about their mother's murder. For decades Sal had kept the police report but had never opened the envelope. Often Sal would put the envelope on the nightstand of whatever dorm or shelter they were living in, alongside a pint of Jack Daniels. "It made it feel like she was closer to me. And Jack, well, you know." You do know, but now is not the time for that.

Sal would never say exactly if they witnessed the murder but over time, before the envelope arrived, you were able to glean enough detail to make the PTSD diagnosis anyway and offer appropriate medications, which were politely refused. Often Sal would miss appointments, and you sent your brief reports to the employer hoping Sal could keep the job, stop drinking, and come back to see this through.

"Would you let me bring in that thing?" Sal finally asked. "Would you open the package? Would you read it?" It seemed therapeutic, so you agree thinking Sal wanted you to read it together. "I've dealt with worse," you think, but barely.

"I just have one question," Sal asks of you. Sal's lively dark eyes flatten and you reach out with a steadying hand. You don't want to know the answer to this question but you have already promised.

So you schedule another appointment. You make a plan. Together you will move carefully. You know all about survivor guilt and trauma. You've been doing this for years.

Sal dropped off the manila envelope at the reception desk and never came back.

And now it's yours. As long as there are people like you, no one ever dies. And the envelope goes into a box and the box goes into a pile and the pile grows larger, and you now move it into the barn along with ratty prayer shawls and tiny bottles of dried-up ink and framed drawings from another time. Menorahs from other countries, Scrabble tiles bouncing along the floorboards, children's scribbles, costume jewelry. Photographs of strangers. Your father's unfinished novels. It's like magical thinking, this pretense that you have some gift to keep things alive.

You don't remember what you thought you would say to Sal about what you read.

But then, you didn't have to.

---

**NINA GABY,** a writer, visual artist, and psychiatric nurse practitioner, spent years hunkered down across from the longest floating bridge east of the Mississippi, maintaining a clinical practice from her kitchen counter while finishing a memoir. Gaby has recently moved back to her upstate New York hometown. Her artwork is held in the Smithsonian, Arizona State University, and the Rochester Institute of Technology.

# My Favorite Patient

SARAH HARVIN

My favorite patient may have been
                                                                       A racist.
His first night, I helped him bathe and shave in his tiny dark room.
My most patient patient showered me with pleases and thank yous.
                                                                       A racist.
His tender wounds smarted as I mopped the blood around the bandages.
My most patient patient showered me with pleases and thank yous.
Bulbous drains hung from stitched holes in his abdomen, bouncing gently as we ambled.

His tender wounds smarted as I mopped the blood around the bandages.
He requested a prayer and we clasped hands: mine brown, his white.
Bulbous drains hung from stitched holes in his abdomen, bouncing gently as we ambled.

I wheeled him out in his only t-shirt, emblazoned with the flag of Dixie.

He requested a prayer and we clasped hands: mine brown, his white.

His first night, I helped him bathe and shave in his tiny dark room.

I wheeled him out in his only t-shirt, emblazoned with the flag of Dixie.

My favorite patient may have been

...A racist

---

**SARAH HARVIN** is a fourth-year medical student at the University of Michigan who plans to apply to a family medicine residency. She received her MS in narrative medicine from Columbia University in 2020. Her academic interests include the role of bias and miscommunication in maternal morbidity and the provision of holistic health care to medical students and trainees. She is passionate about using narrative to bridge the gap between medicine, personal experience, and patient care.

ESSAY

# Untarnished

ALI RIZVI

"Do you abuse your wife?"

I was finishing the electronic health record entry at the end of a thirty-minute office visit and was about to pick up the laptop to exit the exam room. The unusual, unexpected question from the patient caught me completely off-guard. *I think he is trying to be humorous*, I thought to myself.

Unsure of what he meant, I hesitated in replying. "Ahmm, what do you mean, Mr. H?" He repeated the question with a louder enunciation and prolonged emphasis on *ABU-U-USE*.

"Nowadays one hears so much about these Moslem men abusing their wives and children," he added, as if attempting to explain the reason behind his inquiry to be a rather genuine curiosity stemming from his limited understanding of prevailing notions and assumptions.

"Well, what has that got to do with me?" I retorted, implying that perhaps I wasn't really Muslim. I suppose my knee-jerk reaction was to bring to my defense my own convictions (or lack of them) as a self-styled agnostic and freethinker, therefore implying apologetically, *that may be true, but you've got the wrong guy*. (Hindsight note to self: A more appropriate response would have been, "Mr. H, I don't think it is appropriate to discuss such matters during a medical office visit. Why don't we focus today on how we can improve your diabetes management?" Or perhaps, without being defensive, to engage with him more and explore where he was coming from.)

Before I could think of anything further, Mr. H immediately responded with a follow-up question. "But I thought you had mentioned once that you *were* Moslem."

*I don't know where he is going with this*, I thought to myself, getting a little uncomfortable with his line of questioning and still looking for a suitable way of handling the situation. I had no recollection of ever discussing my religious beliefs with Mr. H, but evidently he thought otherwise.

A flurry of confusing thoughts drifted through my mind: This patient had driven ninety-nine miles each way to see me for over a decade, so I'm sure he must like me as his doctor, *right*? He was just being inquisitive—I'm sure my background or origin didn't matter to him, he knew I was a good doctor, and his curiosity was getting the best of him . . . he was probably just getting swept away by what he encountered in the news and discussions on TV, etc.—besides, I couldn't recall ever discussing my ethnicity or affiliation with any of my patients, especially since I considered myself lacking any strong traditional beliefs.

My besieged brain, trying to fend off this onslaught of guilt-by-association, kept trying to come up with answers to exculpate and distance myself from my background. Gazing at the floor to try to convey an erudite and philosophical air, I answered rather deliberately, "Well, see, I was born to parents who were Muslim, but that doesn't mean that I follow the same . . . ahmm . . . I mean . . ." I could sense my answer deteriorating into a cowering and unintelligible blabber.

Primitive defense mechanisms started operating in my head. *Still not able to summon the courage? You need to put Mr. H in his place! Like, Shut up, you bigot! Why are you suddenly asking me all these questions?*

Of course, I said no such thing.

Instead, reaching for the doorknob and anxious to end this uncomfortable conversation, I attempted to flee the examination room to the security of the nursing station but was stopped short by another question.

"Well, what *are* you, then?" It was beginning to feel like an interrogation.

I released a long sigh and tried to collect myself for a moment. Not wanting to ignore or evade the patient's questioning any longer, I turned around to face Mr. H, this time staring directly at him. He had been almost motionless this entire time, sitting smugly in his chair with his legs outstretched in front of him and his hands clasped over his abdomen. I sat down, drew my swivel stool closer to him, and rested my chin on both hands. "Mr. H, I'm just a human being trying to do the best I can for you."

Evidently, Mr. H was not done yet. "So you're not a *jihadi* who wants to kill people and blow up buildings?" His eyebrows furrowed a little as he asked the question, and the corners of his mouth pulled up slightly, as if his face was trying to break into an imperceptible and wry smirk.

*Does he really mean that?* I thought. *Is he serious, or is he trying to be sarcastic and funny?* After all, it does appear to be "open season," and he could conceivably get away with either intention without getting called out by the wizards of political correctness. *Has his perception of me changed overnight from the competent, caring, and trustworthy physician of the last ten years to a bloodthirsty, ideology-driven, and brainwashed criminal?* Worse, being utterly unprepared for this relentless assault, I had unwittingly gone into a defense mode (*It's okay for you to suspect me, but I'm not really one of those people*). In the court of Mr. H's opinion, his own clinician and a well-respected academician had to prove himself as a citizen in good standing. *But surely this was not like Mr. H*, I thought—an educated "gentleman" who was always well dressed, civil, and courteous.

"I don't know. I'm just a human being who is trying to do his best, Mr. H . . ." was all I could muster. I smiled softly at him and stepped out of the room.

I could not get the interaction with Mr. H out of my mind for the rest of the day. Driving back home, I decided to stop and swim a few laps at my local YMCA. It gave me some time to recoil from and reflect on the experience, while struggling with what, if anything, to do next.

That night I addressed the following letter to the patient:

*Dear Mr. H,*

*This letter is in regard to your office visit on January 6. We discussed management of your diabetes, and I gave you additional written suggestions for improving your glucose level and general health.*

*However, because of comments that came from you at the end of the visit, which were directed to me personally and were unrelated to your medical care, I feel that a healthy patient–physician relationship cannot continue. Therefore, this letter serves as notice that my office has decided to terminate its provision of health care to you. We will continue to provide the usual services to you for one month from your receiving this note, or until you are transferred into the care of another physician for the medical issues our office has helped you with.*

*The nature and contents of your remarks that have caused me to make this decision have not been documented in your medical record or elsewhere. They have not been brought to the knowledge of any other person. They remain confidential, and my preference is to maintain privacy unless their revelation becomes necessary or inevitable.*

*I wish you good health in the future.*

The next morning, my secretary typed up the letter and placed it in the inbox for my signature.

Over the next two weeks I took care of all sorts of paperwork—refill authorizations, notes from other physicians, laboratory results—the "stuff" that a clinician normally encounters in a busy medical practice. During all that time, Mr. H's letter sat in the inbox while the rest of the paperwork came and went. I would glance at it only to pick it up and put it back down.

One morning in the clinic, while I was finishing up seeing a patient and was about to go into the next examination room, the nurse pulled me aside and said, "Mr. H's wife called. He started having abdominal pains three days ago and they had to admit him to the hospital. He is passing blood in his stool. They think he might have diverticulitis. His sugars have been running high and they want to adjust his insulin regimen. He is telling them he already has a diabetes doctor and is refusing to make any changes unless they run it by you first. He wants you to call him."

My mind wandered to our conversation at the end of his last office visit. "Okay, tell Mrs. H I will call within the hour," I replied. "Also, I will need to see him for a follow-up appointment within a week after he leaves the hospital," I added with a little hesitation.

Back at my desk at the end of the day, as I was finishing paperwork, my eyes fell on the letter I had written to Mr. H two weeks earlier. It was still on my desk awaiting my signature. I started thinking about my conversation with his wife earlier in the day, and how distraught she was—and yet it was so uplifting for me. "He has been asking for you every day he has been in the hospital. Dr. Rizvi, you know he just doesn't trust anyone else but you when it comes to his sugars," she had said. "Remember when you talked to his family doc about getting him a stress test? He thinks you saved his life. He says you're the only doctor who calls him at home to discuss his test results. You've helped him so much over the years. He sings your praises all the time!" I could not wrap my head around what Mr. H had been saying to his wife about me, especially in view of his line of questioning during his last office visit. *He was confused when he saw me*, I thought to myself. *Perhaps he was only responding to what the media and "opinion pundits" were feeding him—and struggling with categorizing and stereotyping all human beings, including his physician.* We were obviously failing as a society in this respect, and he was one of the victims. Seeds of hatred and division were being sown. A sacred doctor–patient relationship—along with many other bonds in our communities—was being destroyed. I sat back in my chair and thought, *It is okay to understand and forgive.* My sense of commitment to Mr. H's welfare as his healer took precedence over any feelings of anger and resentment, however justifiable, I was harboring. I had the option to ignore and move on.

At that moment, I picked up the letter I had written to Mr. H and glanced at it for a split second. Then I ran it through the shredder.

---

**ALI RIZVI** is a professor of medicine at the University of Central Florida College of Medicine and staff endocrinologist at the VA Medical Center in Orlando. Rizvi, who has been involved in patient care, teaching, mentoring, and research, has also served as chief of endocrinology, endowed professor, and fellowship program director at the University of South Carolina. He enjoys family time, running, swimming, and hiking.

ESSAY

# Bruised Apples

JACK COULEHAN

A MANILA FOLDER labeled "Michael" lies in the bottom drawer of my filing cabinet, along with "Bathroom Renovations" and "1980 Honda," remnants of a time when files were objects that occupied space and gradually turned yellow. The hump in the folder consists of a handful of letters; the last one, written on peculiar blue stationery, is dated September 2, 1981. In it, my friend Michael O'Leary, a registered nurse, apologizes for his behavior. He tells me his mother has had a stroke, and he has come home from California to take care of her. "Right middle cerebral," he writes. "Massive." Paralyzed and dumb. His father is paralyzed too, with grief and dread. "My life is shit," Michael complains.

He writes with his characteristic looping penmanship and wide margins filled with zigzags, stars, and exclamation points. He is overwhelmed by his parents' needs, his brother's indifference.

"My goddamn headaches are back again. I can't get rid of them. Sunlight drives me crazy. I mope around all day. Help!" In the last paragraph he comes to the point: "What I need is some Dilaudid. Could you write me a script for Dilaudid?"

The letter was addressed to my office at the University of Pittsburgh, where the moment I read it I exploded. It's difficult to remember how emotion feels but easy to recall its name and my behavior. Righteous indignation. Swearing. Dashing off an abruptly dismissive note. Tearing it up. Stomping out.

There was another bombshell on the evening news that same night. Michael O'Leary had drowned in the Youghiogheny River. His body was found in the rocky shallows about a half mile beyond the rapids at Ohiopyle. Police speculated that he must have been swimming in the river when he had a seizure. A terrible accident.

As far as I knew, Mike had never learned to swim.

---

The last time I had seen Mike was early on a muggy summer morning three years earlier. I had driven him to the Greyhound bus station in Pittsburgh, after insisting the night before that he leave my house. We didn't say much. When he climbed onto the San Francisco bus, I stood there blankly, barricaded against compassion, determined that he had violated my trust. Good riddance, I told the steering wheel on the way home.

Mike was a high school friend, one of fifteen boys in our tiny class. He was angular, acne-scarred, and when manic the funniest person I've ever known. He and Bill Barnes and I invented the Supreme Council, which secretly ran the universe, and made ourselves its officers. Had this been the '90s instead of the '60s, we would have been considered nerds, but at that time there wasn't any label for us, other than unpopular. After graduation Mike joined the Marines, where he trained to be a medic. They sent him to Vietnam, where he experienced the heart of darkness for two years. Later, he became a nurse.

I'd see Mike occasionally during medical school, but later, when my wife and I lived on the Navajo reservation in the early '70s, we were within striking distance of his home base at Merced in California's Central Valley. He worked in a migrant workers' clinic run by a clutch of hippie doctors who lived in a commune. When we visited Mike, we talked politics, injustice, the Vietnam War, and especially the plight of migrant farm workers. Mike damned the federal government, while ignoring the fact that I was employed by the same warmongers, possibly because he considered caring for Native Americans a worthwhile endeavor, even under questionable auspices. In any case, at Mike's house we were able to let our hair down—listen to music, smoke pot, and argue all night. He called himself our "social director," clueing us in to folk singers and rock bands he relished. Each time we visited him we came home with stacks of old LPs, like *Joy of Cooking* and Phil Ochs and the Beatles' *White Album*. Mike had a huge American flag that he used as a throw on his living room sofa. It gave him a lot of satisfaction to sit on the flag, despite the fact the Marines had paid for his education. I still have a photograph of our diaper-less eight-month-old son sitting happily on the Stars and Stripes after having peed prodigiously. It made for a hilarious story.

Mike was wild. Girlfriends came and went. He moved to the coast for a while. The next thing we heard he had driven to Nicaragua and was working at a rural clinic there, twelve hours a day, seven days a week. So much work. So little time. And then back to the San Joaquin Valley. After a while we heard about his breakdown, his diagnosis, his stint as an inpatient at the San Diego VA Hospital. I think it was his latest girlfriend who kept us informed. Michael was doing well, she wrote. Better. Always better. She was a lovely woman.

We were living in Pittsburgh when Mike showed up on our porch one day with his duffel bag and asked to stay for a while. After the breakdown, he was stronger, a new man, he explained, and back on his own two feet. I'd never seen him so high and scattered and brittle as he was then, clearly manic. He said he needed just a little help. Could I become his doctor?

First, there were his headaches. Like me, Mike had been a migraineur since high school. This was in the days before effective migraine-specific treatment existed, although in his case it probably didn't matter. In fact, he had started to take opioids early and often, although in the Merced days I wasn't aware of it. Somehow, he managed to get a steady supply of Dilaudid.

Or at least he did until lithium straightened him out. Now I'm fine, he said. I'm stable. My mood is good. No more dope. It's just that the headaches have come back. I need something.

Dilaudid. Just a little.

We took him in. He planned to get a job. He hadn't seen his parents in years and intended to visit them. He had never met his brother's wife or seen his nephew. He would start job hunting first thing the next morning. Maybe he did, but by early afternoon Mike arrived at the community clinic where I worked and asked the receptionist for an appointment.

You're crazy, I told him. I can't see you. Just pretend you don't know me, he said. I need your help. I can't talk now, I told him. I have to go. Come back at five. I'll give you a ride home.

He pestered me for a week about this. In the process he told me his story, the ups and downs, the manic psychosis, the drug rehab. In between the bouts of nagging, Mike was his usual hilarious self. My wife and I stayed on edge much of the time, but just when we approached the limit Mike did something sensitive or generous, like sending her a bunch of red roses. I broke down and wrote him a script for lithium when he promised me that he had made a psych appointment at the Pittsburgh VA. However, when the time came, it slipped his mind, or he wasn't feeling well that morning. Finally, after he had stayed in bed for two days with his face in the pillow because of a migraine, I wrote him a script for Dilaudid. Ten tablets. Of course, I wanted to make it official, so I took him to the clinic and examined him and set up a medical record. I think the clinic even tried to bill Medicaid in California. But none of these measures diminished my guilt about being manipulated. After the second Dilaudid prescription, I drew the line.

Following the Dilaudid confrontation, Mike got louder, more raucous. He also became more obsessive about the book he was supposedly writing, an exposé of incompetence in the VA. For several days we couldn't tell whether Mike would come down from the spare room and disrupt our evening by chasing the children around until they became cranky or stay in his room in front of his typewriter and stare into the distance. After a week of this I told him he had to go. He cried and promised and promised and cried but then gave up and called his girlfriend and made arrangements to return to San Francisco. The next morning I drove him to the bus.

The letter's postmark is dated three days before they found his body, discovered by picnickers spending a pleasant Sunday afternoon along the river. According to the news, Mike had been in the water at least twenty-four hours. He must have jumped from the highway bridge, or somehow forced himself to walk into a deep pool of the river, like Virginia Woolf. I guess suicide wasn't mentioned out of respect for his family and to allow his burial in sacred ground. I went to the wake that Monday after work, to the town at the base of Laurel Ridge, where Mike and I used to spend our weekends hiking and fooling around. One summer we found a geological map in the public library of all the caves along the ridge and spent weeks spelunking the lot of them. In our Supreme Council meetings, we discussed plans for improving the world.

The first thing we intended to do was outlaw nuns. The second thing Mike had in mind was to arrest the rich people who lived at the end of his street and give their big white house to his parents.

What I remember about the wake is Michael's despondent father. He was a small man who had always seemed colorless because he was neither a big shot nor an intellectual, but drove a bakery truck. He hovered beside the casket, which was nestled among a dozen flower arrangements, including one with white lilies from California that had in gold letters across it ALL MY LOVE, BABE. Many of my high school friends were there. We talked on the porch, but none of them invited me to go out later for a drink.

After all, it had been more than twenty years.

    Instead of driving home, I stayed at the Motel 6 that night. The apple orchard beside the motel may still have belonged to the people who lived in the big house that Mike coveted so much. Inside my room, spores from the air conditioner replaced the sweet smell of rotting apples that pervaded the parking lot. Before going to bed, I went out and walked through the orchard, up one row and down another, again and again, unintentionally mashing some of the fallen, bruised apples. There were so many of them, and it was a moonless night.

---

**JACK COULEHAN** is an emeritus professor of preventive, family, and population medicine at Stony Brook University's Renaissance School of Medicine. Coulehan's essays, poems, and stories appear frequently in health care journals, literary magazines, and anthologies. He is the author of seven poetry collections, including *The Talking Cure: New and Selected Poems*.

ESSAY

# Dr. Ortega and the Fajita Man

RICHARD B. WEINBERG

"Oh, no! Not again!" moaned the endoscopy fellow upon answering his pager in the middle of GI grand rounds.

"Fajita Man?" someone ventured.

"Yeah, Mr. Gutierrez is back in the ED again with another food impaction! I'll go get the travel cart," he said dejectedly. "Who's the attending on call today?"

By now, everyone in our GI section knew Mr. Gutierrez quite well. He was a ninety-one-year-old widower from Oaxaca who had come to live with his son. Aside from moderate dementia and having no teeth, he was otherwise in good health, with the exception of a distal esophageal stricture that had defied attempts at endoscopic dilation. As long as Mr. Gutierrez followed a mechanical soft diet, all was well. But he did not do that.

With increasing frequency, after his son left for work, Mr. Gutierrez would wander the barrio in search of a restaurant that served his favorite food: fajitas. There he would savor his forbidden meal until his esophagus was packed to the top with unmasticated meat, at which point he would start to choke. A 911 call, an ambulance ride to our ED, and a stat page to the GI fellow on call would ensue. This was becoming a monthly event.

As the months went by, the hospital administration became increasingly frustrated and concerned because Mr. Gutierrez was uninsured and our endoscopic services were costing the hospital thousands of dollars in unreimbursed expenses. They sent a social worker to visit his home, but she reported back that Mr. Gutierrez was well cared for by his son and appeared to be quite happy; otherwise, she had no brilliant ideas about how to stop his fajita forays. "Do something!" the administration implored the GI section.

So we arranged a meeting with Mr. Gutierrez's son. He told us he had tried to stop his father from wandering off by locking the doors whenever he was not at home and even by hiring a sitter to watch him, but to no avail. "He can escape anything and anyone, just like Ayala," he told us, referring to the famous Mexican illusionist who some compared to Houdini. "He's got dentures, but he refuses to wear them, and begging him to stop eating fajitas is useless, because he can't remember what happens when he eats them, let alone what I say from one minute to the next. And I can't cut off his money, because he's squirrelled away cash all over the house." Everyone was at a loss.

The next time Mr. Gutierrez appeared in the ED I was fortunate to be on call with the chief GI fellow, Carlos Francisco Ortega III, MD. A third-generation Hispanic physician, Dr. Ortega radiated a magnetic bonhomie that instantly made him everybody's best friend. Even as a resident, he looked like a prosperous private practitioner. He dressed impeccably, sported a large gold class ring, and drove a BMW M6, which he parked off-site, lest our section head see a GI fellow driving a car that was much more expensive than his own. Dr. Ortega also proved to be an intuitively skilled endoscopist from the first day of his fellowship. In facing a fajita-filled esophagus, there was no one I would rather have standing by my side than Dr. Ortega (to tell the truth, I stood by his).

"¡Hola Señor Gutierrez!" Dr. Ortega warmly greeted our recurrent patient, accompanied by his son, at his bedside. "¿Comiste fajitas otra vez?" (Did you eat fajitas again?), he asked gently.

"Sí, pero no están bajando" (Yes, but they aren't going down),

Mr. Gutierrez replied, somewhat bewildered.

"No te preocupes. Te vamos a arreglar." (Don't worry. We're going to fix you.)

Sedation administered and scope in hand, "¡Traga!" (Swallow!), Dr. Ortega exhorted, easily passed the endoscope, and set to work.

Without recounting the gross technical details, let me assure you that of all the foods that can cause an esophageal impaction, fajitas are the worst. They are stringy, slippery, and frustratingly elusive to even the cleverest endoscopic foreign body removal device. A fajita disimpaction can take hours.

Nonetheless, given Dr. Ortega's skill, we cleared Mr. Gutierrez's esophagus in record time.

Once Mr. Gutierrez had awakened from sedation, in a vain attempt to discern the reason behind his repeated fajita transgressions, I asked Dr. Ortega to question him.

"Señor Gutierrez, why do you keep eating fajitas?" Dr. Ortega inquired in Spanish. Mr. Gutierrez's exuberant reply made Dr. Ortega laugh out loud. "He says it's because they taste good! They're his favorite food!" Mr. Gutierrez nodded and smiled toothlessly.

Dr. Ortega chatted a bit more with Mr. Gutierrez and his son in rapid, animated Spanish, but he did not bother to translate the conversation for me. "I've got an idea," he remarked as we were packing up the travel cart to return to the endoscopy unit.

Sometime later that year I was staffing an emergency consult in the ED with Dr. Ortega and casually remarked that no one had seen Mr. Gutierrez for months.

"Oh, I don't think he'll be coming back anymore," he opined coyly.

"Why? Did he die?"

"No, I fixed the problem. After we did his last endoscopy, I asked him what his other favorite foods were. He told me that after fajitas, his favorite foods are dessert sweets like flan, jericalla, and arroz con leche. I know his neighborhood pretty well, so one weekend I visited all the restaurants and food vendors within a ten-mile radius of his house and gave them posters I printed up with a photo of him and the warning:

> "*If you see this man* DO NOT SERVE HIM FAJITAS!
>
> "*He is allergic to meat, and* HE WILL DIE! *Offer him a soft dessert sweet instead, and call his son at 281-555-0154.*"

"You gotta be kidding! That actually worked?" I asked incredulously.

"As far as I know, he hasn't been back to the ED since. I visited him a couple of times to check up on him. He's doing just fine. I brought him some of my mother's flan de naranja, which he loves. He's really a charming old man—he reminds me of my abuelo."

"This is beyond belief, Carlos! Have you told anyone else about this?"

"No, not yet. I wanted to make sure it worked first."

"Well, maybe it's time!"

When word finally circulated around the hospital about how Dr. Ortega "cured" the Fajita Man of his troublesome affliction, he became an instant legend. The ED staff presented him with a plaque that read *World's Greatest Gastroenterologist*; the internal medicine house staff voted him Clinician of the Year, and the hospital administration arranged a special dinner at a five-star hotel for the entire GI section as a token of their gratitude.

The evening was a grand affair, with a cocktail reception and a four-course sit-down dinner. We were not entirely surprised to see that the main course was fajitas.

---

**RICHARD B. WEINBERG** is a professor of gastroenterology and internal medicine at Wake Forest University School of Medicine and the Graduate School of Biomedical Sciences. A graduate of the

Johns Hopkins University School of Medicine and the University of Chicago internal medicine and gastroenterology training programs, Weinberg, who has been an academic physician for over five decades, has written extensively about the transformational impact of the doctor–patient relationship.

# 3

# THE SOUND AND THE FURIES

*Shame and Anger*

SHORT STORY

# Old Scrubs

BRUCE H. CAMPBELL

Dr. Hal Winters remembers watching construction workers pour and grind the terrazzo floors in this wing of the hospital. Over the three decades since then, he has walked these corridors thousands of times; each crack, patch, and undulation is familiar. Were there ever a need to get from one end of the building to the other in pitch darkness—during a power failure or natural disaster, perhaps—he could find his way by tracing the floor's subtle ripples and feeling the textures and seams of the wall coverings. *Someday, before I retire, I'll try doing just that.* He turns the corner and heads toward the operating room as efficiently as his aging joints will allow.

Hal's patient, Betty, is half asleep by the time he changes into scrubs and walks into OR25. Over the years, he has biopsied, removed, or reconstructed something on nearly every member of Betty's family. He grips her shoulder. "We'll have that big old lump out of your neck in a jiffy! I'll talk to Cliff as soon as we're done. See you in Recovery." She nods as her eyelids drift closed. In a few minutes, the procedure is underway.

Hal pulls the knife through the skin and begins to separate the normal tissues from the rock-hard mass. "Retractor." He rearranges the instruments. "Here, hold this," he says to the surgical tech. Hal notices that the mass is stuck to the surrounding muscles and veins. *This is going to be more difficult than I thought.*

The chief of surgery, Dr. Julie Pembroke, peeks through the doorway. "Good morning, everyone!" she sings. "Everything okay, Dr. Winters?"

Hal glances up, squinting obliquely at her from under his heavy, graying eyebrows. Back in the day, when Dr. Pembroke was probably still in high school, Hal was working eighty hours per week and tackling every challenge thrown at him. Colleagues referred their most difficult cases. Not anymore. No one said anything, but he knows people call the younger surgeons now. He pauses, shrugs, and drops his gaze back to the surgical field. "Got it covered, Doctor. Thank you." There is an unmistakable growl in his voice. Her face disappears and the door drifts closed.

Soon, the mass is almost out. As his knife makes its final swipe, blood unexpectedly floods the operative field. "More sponges!" He instinctively presses his left fingertips firmly into the center of the wound, stanching the flow of blood pouring from the vein he has inadvertently cut. "I need you to pay attention!" he barks at the surgical tech. "Unclamp the suction!" She reaches to release the suction tubing. "Now give me another hemostat!" He plunges the tips of the clamp into the pooling blood, aiming where, experience tells him, the vein has been damaged. He tightens the clamp and tilts its handle toward the tech. "Here, steady this while I tie things off." He throws some knots, then removes the hemostat from the wound. The bleeding resumes unchecked. "Another clamp!" He repeats the process twice, adding more ties. He throws stitches into the wound and snugs the sutures tight. "All right," he says. "Let's see if that did it." He releases pressure on the wound and watches. The bleeding is controlled. "Okay. That's better. Let's get this thing closed."

Hal rinses the wound with saline and dries the area with a gauze. As he does so, he notices an unexpected glistening, pale, spaghetti-noodle-sized white stump of tissue caught in one of his silk ties. "Damn," he says. "Get me a nerve stimulator." Hal reluctantly touches the electrode of the device to the stump, then groans as the nearby muscles jump vigorously. *Just what I needed,* he thinks. *I cut the damn nerve.* "Call someone from Plastics and tell them to come fix this."

Ninety minutes later, the young plastic surgeon—whose name Hal has forgotten—is giving her contact information to Betty's husband. "Now, Clifford," she warns, "even though we sewed the cut ends of the nerve back together, her range of motion will never be the same. Her shoulder muscles will be very weak for several months so physical therapy will be critical. Make an appointment to see me next week." Hal wonders how quickly news of his complication is spreading through the hospital. He avoids Cliff's gaze and says little.

Betty is sitting up in bed when Hal stops by the recovery room. He grips her hand for a few seconds, frowns, then heads to the locker room, avoiding the surgeons' lounge and the OR front desk.

The locker room is empty when Hal sits down on the bench and kicks off his old, stained surgical shoes. He pulls off his scrubs and dresses slowly.

After dropping his scrubs in the laundry hamper, Hal slips into his lab coat. He grabs his pager off the locker shelf, clips it to his belt, then pats his pockets to make certain he has not left anything behind. He hears the hospital-issue lock bang against the chipped blue painted metal as he kicks the locker door closed. He looks around the room and turns to leave.

People push past Hal as he makes his way into the brightly lit corridor. After two tentative steps, he brushes the fingertips of his right hand against the wall, gathers in a deep breath, and continues silently down the long, familiar hallway with his eyes tightly closed.

---

**BRUCE H. CAMPBELL** is a retired head and neck cancer surgeon, narrative medicine enthusiast, essayist, and author of *A Fullness* *of Uncertain Significance: Stories of Surgery, Clarity, and Grace.* He lives near Milwaukee, Wisconsin. Find more of his work at BruceCampbellMD.com.

ESSAY

# Black Tango

PHILIP BERRY

ON EVERY WARD round he looks up (though I try to meet his gaze from an equal height, sitting on the bed) and finds the positives. He presumes there is a surgical cure, though I know already that it cannot be. He welcomes the idea of chemotherapy—it worked so well last time—but I know it can offer nothing more than a brief extension.

He is forty-eight. He lives on hope as the fatally undermined airplane flies on fumes, its passengers observing the steady passage of the clouds in deep, sweet ignorance. I believe the face he wears to meet the face of his wife, that "we can deal with this" mask, can be fixed by no other kind of glue. He thinks she needs to hear that there is a future, so his mind cannot admit of any alternative. That is my amateur psychological analysis. But I have seen her leaving the cubicle, how the thin smile straightens as she turns away into the outside world, and I think she knows. She does not know the facts, but she recognizes death in her husband's sunken features.

I am too negative. The modern way is never to say there is no hope, that "nothing can be done." There are many things we can do, there is much we can offer. Palliative care is a specialty in itself, a branch of medicine as established now as cardiology or oncology. We *will* treat you.

Yes, yes, yes, of course you will. But you can't *save* me, can you? They see through our pretense. Come on! When you're forty-eight and dying of cancer, you don't want to hear how great the palliative care is. Do you?

I don't know. I'm not dying.

The problem with this chap is, he's been through it before. This is a recurrence. In another hospital, at a preposterously young age, he got pancreatic cancer. Another hospital, another country, another hemisphere in fact. They did a good job, technically. Cut out the tumor, replaced a major abdominal vein with a graft, re-plumbed an adjacent artery. When I read the op notes (lifted from his impeccably kept folder) I sighed. It must have been edging into those vessels. Locally advanced, as we say. And far too many nodes. Of the seven they removed, six contained cancer. But they hammered him with chemo, cleaned the circuits of any rogue cells, got him through a few bouts of neutropenia, and gave him the all-clear. Cured.

He was never cured.

It was bound to return. Ask any pancreatic surgeon, they will shake their head. Locally advanced, nodal spread. Borrowed time.

He was not aware. He had been feeling odd for two or three months now, and it did not occur to him that it might have come back. Even now, in this hospital, he seems not to know that so manifest a recurrence of symptoms (he is jaundiced, the cancer is blocking off his liver) can mean only one thing.

I want to ring that highly skilled surgeon on the other side of the world and ask him (I read the op note, it's a he): What were you playing at, letting him think he was cured? Didn't you know what the prognosis was? You let him go back to his family, change jobs, live his life, with no idea that what is happening now was *inevitable*. All the plans he made, all the images he entertained. False. All false. Built on a foundation of lies. No, not lies, that's too strong. Just the absence of truth. You let the best-case scenario flower into a confirmed reality. And now it's crashing down around him.

If I ever see him—in some sunny pancreatic conference, on

some doctor-packed airplane—I will tell him this directly. Look at the mess you left for me to clear up. Me. For it is I who must now sit with him, tomorrow, perhaps next week, when all the facts are in place and all the opinions have been given, to dismantle the delicate construction that occupies his deluded mind. That high tower around which winged visions flutter and speak of future milestones, his daughter's next birthday party, the work that needs to be done on the house, that second home.

Future life. A life which I, the messenger, must now take away.

The messenger. Brings to mind a line from *Antony and Cleopatra*. I saw it last week. Ralph Fiennes was the lead. The messenger, quaking, comes to tell the Egyptian queen that her love has betrayed her in taking a wife. "I that do bring the news made not the match," he says, to Cleopatra's threat that the bearer of bad news "shalt be whipp'd with wire, and stew'd in brine, Smarting in lingering pickle." A good night it was. My wife's hand lay in mine, both of us enjoying a rare excursion. A good life, a London life, privileged. Why do I tell you this? Because as I sat there, before the spectacle, he, the He of this piece, floated across my field of vision from stage left. Lying in bed, yellow with jaundice, his face tense with pain, smarting from the puncture that my colleagues in radiology had made in his side to drain the bile ducts. That's how I left him on Friday night, before throwing on my scarf and heading off to the theater. I left him waiting for morphine.

I know the *how*. There will be a specialist nurse, hopefully an oncologist too. I will compress his future between my honest hands using carefully chosen words laced in maximum empathy. We will advise that he has four to six months with chemo or two, maybe less, without. (I wouldn't take that deal, personally.) We will remain positive, talking of all that can be done. He will see through it. Then I will watch the mask begin to crumble, like a petrified monster tapped by the hero's sword, falling away to form a pile of gray powder on the floor.

What about the *when*? Tomorrow. I have danced around it for too long. There are no more behind-the-scenes negotiations to be had. The multidisciplinary team meeting has reached its consensus—no surgery, no cure. Every hour that passes without honest communication adds to the deceit. We know what he does not. Have known, for days. Since before the play, to be honest.

There have been whispered conversations outside the bay. Yesterday the nurse in charge of the ward asked me, "Have you discussed resuscitation status?" No. NO! That comes later, after I have confirmed to him there is no cure. Be patient. But it is a sign. He looks bad now, his energy is failing. The nurses' senses are attuned to the possibility of sudden crisis. It has gone on for too long, this black tango. It cannot be allowed to continue.

―

I sat with them and talked, but they knew everything. I told them nothing they did not already know.

It was I who walked in the dark.

He saw me dancing with words, he read my evasions, and he waited. Waited until I was ready.

He was protecting me, the messenger. And he was kind. Too kind.

---

**PHILIP BERRY** is a consultant hepatologist and clinical director at St. Thomas' Hospital in London. He writes on medical ethics, end-of-life care, and the welfare of health care workers. He is the author of *Necessary Scars: A Doctor's Life in Error*.

POEM

# Kübler-Ross

S. K. RANCY

First
there was despair :
I thought
I would drown & choke
on my own tears, thought
my tongue would burn
forever
with their perditious salt

Then came
rage : violent
tumultuous
the way waves devour
each other, the way
Jacob wrestled
with an Angel at Peniel,
pinning back
Its glorious downy wings

so that he might

break Its back—

so I wrestled with my soul (if

it truly shimmers

there, beneath the skin)

and so I wrestled

with God

The rage

has not quite

      flown

           away

nor has

the despair .

---

**S. K. RANCY** is a Haitian American poet, novelist, and surgical resident in New York City. A graduate of Columbia University, his poetry has appeared in *Apogee Journal*, *Moko*, *Sargasso*, and *Seventh Wave*. His books include the poetry collection *Dreams of Diaspora* and the poetry chapbook *Self-Portrait in Hospital as Camus*.

ESSAY

# The Halo

XI CHEN

THE DOCTORS ARE talking. An autumnal blizzard wipes flecks of frost across the windowpane.

"Mr. M—," the younger doctor intones, "is a twenty-five-year-old man with a past medical history significant for chronic alcohol abuse."

The older doctor bows his head and stands with arms crossed, feet together. The older doctor listens intently. Falling snow is a metaphor for words.

"Mr. M—," the younger doctor continues, "presents to the NMICU status post craniotomy day ten for H.H. 2, M.F.G. 3 subarachnoid hemorrhage, and C-1 fracture secondary to recurrent cranial trauma—"

The older doctor interrupts for clarification, and the younger doctor confesses to not having the information. They look at the patient to fill in the silence. I have the information, but I keep my lips sealed.

"Mr. M—," the younger doctor continues, "his hospital course was complicated by persistent vasospasm, refractory to nimo . . . nimodipine prophylaxis and verapamil via D.S.A."

Gray light from the cemetery across the street leaches through the melting frost, which is solidifying into ice. The doctors are talking in hushed, rushed cantos.

I watch with pen and paper. I watch from the entrance to the patient's room, with half of my body in the unit, where there is security in numbers. I watch with a wrinkled pad of lined paper in my hand, not writing down a word. I exist to learn how to speak like them, to learn how to summon a snowstorm in early September.

Besides, I have heard this story before.

The rhythmic beeping of vital signs is our metric of time. The elongated gasps from the ventilator eliminate any possibility of true silence. I bore ink infinities into the paper, like a bored toddler doodling in the pews, and stare out at Mr. M—. My eyelids are heavy, and I cannot maintain a steady gaze. My vision ripples with its own echoes, and a wave of nausea hits my gut.

Mr. M— lays sprawled in his hospital bed, airless and still, surrounded by the language of machines.

There are no family members present to meet with the team. There are traces of them, though: a box of tissues with the cover ripped off. The subtle imprint of a butt on the visitor's chair. A plastic radio gurgling soft jazz. Rings of water on the patient's unused food tray.

This is all a vague illusion, of course. It has been many months since visitors were allowed in the hospital.

I suddenly feel deeply ashamed of being there. For ogling. For Mr. M—'s profound boredom, having to listen to strangers ramble on about his case. This is an absurd feeling, because he is completely snowed.

A nurse replaces a bag of saline as the doctors talk. It occurs to me that Mr. M—'s eyes are just barely open. They are encrusted with dried blood, debris, and ointment. His cheeks and orbits are horribly swollen, but they do not hide the whites of his sclera. They are powerful discs of light; they are powerful refutations of a decaying face.

I cannot turn away from it. There is an intense gravity in the room that only someone as naive as a medical student can sense. It radiates from the increasing entropy of Mr. M—'s body, in its various stages of healing and breakdown. I am struck with an urge to draw it in my notes: the immobile limbs, arranged at unnatural angles, held together by casts and metal rods. Several thin sheets creating their own twisted chaos. Tubes, too many tubes, simultaneously nourishing and cleansing the bloodstream. The chest, grandly exposed, strewn with EKG-leads. The scene is unabashedly sordid, but through my dewy-eyed sight it has an odd holiness. If only I could reach out and change it, tidy the bed, or cover his bare feet . . . but the doctors are still talking.

When the younger doctor finishes, the older doctor—a neurologist who specializes in intensive care—turns to me out of obligation and asks for my brief impressions of the case. I nod gently at Mr. M— and say that I think the case is very sad.

Everyone agrees, so I pass for the day.

There are no family members present to meet with the team, but I suppose it is better that way. The older doctor walks to the head of the bed and begins the physical exam. I'm told this is the crown jewel of neurology, the thoroughness and utility of the physical exam. That neurologists don't rely on lab tests and imaging when they can diagnose with the sheer might of their hands. The hand, the only tool used by humans, gentle enough to cradle a baby and fierce enough to wield a war-hammer.

"Besides," the younger doctor later says to me about the physical exam, "it's free."

It's also overrated, at least in the Neuromedicine Intensive Care Unit (NMICU) setting. A majority of the patients already have clear-cut diagnoses, with the most common being strokes, brain hemorrhages, trauma, and tumors. For the team, doing the exam is less a matter of discovery than a constellation of data points to compare with prior exams. It's an additional metric of recovery, or deterioration.

The neurological exam is also a profound source of stress relief.

The older doctor prefers to start from the top and work his way down. For humans, there is nothing more top than the mind.

I stand in awe as the neurologist places his face within a few inches of Mr. M—'s and bellows the poor man's name over and over again.

For the awake and alert patient, the "mental status exam" generally involves a series of simple questions about one's identity, date of birth, location in space and time, what's this on my wrist called, can you spell the word "world" backwards, etc. The mind is the only function of the nervous system not encased in skin or skull, and thus it can only be accessed by language.

The comatose patient presents a unique challenge, in which the tools used become increasingly more primitive, and violent.

The echoes of Mr. M—'s name fill the unit with an avalanche of sound. One's name is the single word that people will fight to respond to, when said loud enough and with excessive repetition. Against the weight of sedation and delirium, most people will at least flutter their eyes, twitch a muscle, or moan.

It dawns on me that this is medicine's essential task, and the source of its power: to bring language from the realm of the ideas to concrete flesh. When a physician is unable to achieve this lofty goal, this unique sovereignty over broken bodies, they can easily fall into causing language's polar opposite: pain.

A squall shakes the window. The older doctor shines a light into Mr. M—'s eyes.

Disappointed, he begins his game of nociception. The right foot is held in one hand, and tickled with the other. When this fails to trigger spontaneous giggles, the doctor takes his thumb and slowly draws a question mark from Mr. M—'s heel up to the bottom of his big toe. We all watch for the reflexive flaring of the toes known as the plantar reflex. When there is none, he digs his thumb in harder.

In terms of medical necessity, these steps are sufficient. The neurological intensivist often goes further, however, to prove by exhaustion that everything was tried to stimulate the patient's consciousness. The match cannot be forfeited before the king is captured, or until the board falls apart.

Like a medieval knight raising a polearm, the older doctor draws his reflex hammer from the deep recesses of his white coat. The hammer has a weighted mallet for providing a solid and satisfying strike against tendons, but the neurologist instead uses the metal body of the hammer, pressing it down against the nail bed of Mr. M's big toe. No response. He invites me to come try, for educational purposes. Monkey see, monkey do. He warns me to be gentle, lest I be sued for breaking a nail.

There are a seemingly endless number of these mechanical "noxious stimuli." I will list them here. After the reflex hammer is retired, the neurologist begins pinching a variety of muscles, especially those in the legs. We take turns going up to Mr. M— and seizing hunks of his flesh in our fingers. Bruising from previous exams is evident.

Next, the excruciating "trap squeeze" in which the trapezius, a flat and triangular muscle that stretches over the shoulders like a scarf, is grabbed and tortured between the thumb and two fingers.

This is followed by the most universally known noxious stimulus, the "sternal rub," in which a clenched fist is used to dig into the sternum, the blade of bone that defends the heart. This maneuver is sometimes performed for up to thirty seconds.

By far the most painful method, which is like a forbidden spell I have only ever learned of in lectures and books, is the application of supraorbital pressure. The supraorbital notch is a groove in the skull surrounding the eye, two finger-widths lateral to the mid-face, just underneath the eyebrow. Pushing hard on the notch compresses the nerve running through it, which should produce an intense pain localized to the eye and scalp, like a sinus headache.

This is the one technique I have difficulty practicing on myself.

Thus, the older doctor traverses the terrain of Mr. M—'s body, crushing nerves and dispelling perfusion. I begin to write things down.

I can see he wants to go even further. A face mask cannot hide a scowl. Perhaps the older doctor was considering supraorbital pressure, or even a direct blow to Mr. M—'s face.

It is shameful for a doctor to have such thoughts.

Mr. M—'s head is hardly touchable, regardless. It's the first thing one notices when walking into the room: the ring of black metal with long rods extending from its circumference into the patient's scalp. A veritable crown of thorns, holding Mr. M—'s head aloft and, most important, immobile.

A doctor should never give up, but the older doctor cannot help but sigh and slump his shoulders. The surgery had not helped. He walks out of the room. The younger doctor and I follow.

"Let's go write notes," the older doctor says.

---

**XI CHEN** is a resident doctor at NYU Langone Health and a graduate of the Columbia Writing Program, where he received an MFA in creative nonfiction. His essays have appeared in *Literary Hub*, *The Rumpus*, and *The Guardian*.

# Intro to Physicianship

## LALA TANMOY DAS

It is his first graded test on breaking news
—unexpected, the still-

birth, planned perfectly until
the sudden tear in a branch

of arteries—and the racing
heart has stopped underneath

a cage of supple ribs, lips leaking verbs
unspoken, the six-month fetus—

now, a pale blue stillness. He is scored
on the professionalism with which

this tragedy is conveyed—perfect pitch,
narrow wit, optimal empathy, points even

for the right amount of eye contact—
a course on the basics of physicianship.

He conveys with poise; the rubric
of grades checkered in his mind—hiding

the crackle of voice, holding tears back
behind his pale curtain of lids. Later

that night he will come home to me,
sit by my side and scream

hysterically, and I will hold his hand
along the meander of veins, my skin—a raincoat

against the torrent of pain swelling out
from the corners of his lips.

---

**LALA TANMOY (TOM) DAS** is an MD-PhD student at the Weill Cornell Medicine, Rockefeller University, and Memorial Sloan Kettering Cancer Center tri-institutional program in New York City. His writing has appeared in *The New York Times*, *The Washington Post*, *Time* magazine, and *Scientific American*. He lives in New York City with his partner, Eric Kutscher, and their fur baby, Babka.

ESSAY

# Red Line Rising

MICHAEL BROWN

IF YOU COULD walk in my shoes and look through my eyes as I fight in the primary care trenches of America, you might see something like this:

It would begin with a fight between two homeless men, probably over some spare change or a scrap of food, under the I-565 overpass. One of them, a sixty-one-year-old African American male, would get the worst end of the exchange—a fist fit neatly inside the bony orbit of his right eye, his assailant's bare knuckles impacting like a rock from a slingshot.

The concussive force of the blow would send a shock wave through the eye and its crystalline lens, which is about the size and shape of a plain M&M candy. Situated behind the colored tissue of the iris, it captures the light entering the pupil and focuses it onto the macula, the bull's-eye of the retina.

Microscopic cracks and fissures would form, allowing water in the vitreous humor to penetrate the protective lens capsule, flooding its inner core. The sudden intumescence, along with a chain of deleterious metabolic events, would cause the lens to enlarge and opacify, like a milky whitewater balloon.

The lens, waterlogged and heavy, would start to tear away from the zonules, the tiny fibrils that anchor it to the ciliary body at the base of the iris. It would begin to shift forward, blocking the pupil and impeding the flow of aqueous humor from the posterior segment of the eye to the anterior chamber, the space between the iris and the cornea, where, in its angular crevice, the fluid is drained away in the trabecular meshwork, the eye's "sink." The intraocular pressure, normally a delicate balance of tension ranging from 11 to 21 mmHg, would begin to spike.

This shift in stasis would cause the iris to bow forward toward the cornea, further crowding the space where the aqueous drains, causing the pressure to rise even more. The iris would shift forward so much, in fact, it would begin to touch the back surface of the cornea, the clear window of the eye, causing the endothelial "pump" responsible for maintaining the delicate balance of water required for corneal clarity to fail.

The cornea would start to swell too. The rising pressure would force fluid past the normally watertight endothelium and into the laminated middle layers of the stroma, and finally into the outermost epithelium, where tiny blisters would begin to form and erupt.

The pressure would also push backward toward the optic nerve, causing its delicate structure to begin to cave. The retinal nerve fibers, converging to form the optic nerve like the wires in a fiber-optic cable, would begin to fray and atrophy.

As the cataract became denser and the optic nerve more wasted, the homeless man's vision would begin to fade. As the cornea continued to swell and blister, his eye would begin to hurt like hell.

The homeless man would start to make his rounds from ER to ER, begging for pain medication. An ophthalmologist on call at one of them gives him two prescriptions for eye drops and tells him that he needs surgery. He does not give him samples, nor does he admit him.

He has no car, no money, no health insurance, and no way to get the needed medicine. He has even less hope that things are going to turn out even remotely close to well.

Because he is a military veteran, he is eligible for care in your clinic and eventually shows up on your doorstep near the end of the day as you're trying to finish your last two patients. How he got there, and how he found you, nobody knows.

When the primary care physician doing walk-in intake that day dumps him in your lap (you don't blame him), you sigh, plant your face in your palms, and pull down on your skin in an effort to relax your jaw and facial muscles.

You know you're being tested, and you don't want to fail.

You invite the man back to the exam room. You don't think about how he got to be homeless, you don't judge, and you don't ask yourself whether or not he "deserves" care.

He has a disease, he's in pain, you're a doctor, and he's standing there in front of you.

Your duty is clear.

You speak very slowly and plainly, and you observe. You notice there is swelling in the lids and tissue around his right eye and he is holding it as if trying to keep it from popping straight out onto the floor.

But you know the real reason for this universal gesture of distress is he can't stand the glare of your office lights. You dim them as much as possible, and you seat him in your exam chair.

You test his vision in the damaged eye and discover he can barely see the motion of your hand in front of his face. You measure his intraocular pressure and it's 45 mmHg—lower than you thought it would be, but still dangerously high.

You see the milky balloon of a lens, the bulging iris nudging the back surface of the cornea, the painful blisters—hundreds of them.

You diagnose a traumatic cataract with pupillary block glaucoma, but you don't use big words with the patient. You simply tell him his eye pressure is dangerously high and he will likely never see well out of the eye again.

You tell him he might be able to save his eye, and what little vision he has left, if he has surgery. This will require a trip to Birmingham and hospitalization. "But first things first," you say, "let's lower the pressure."

You give him two drops chosen from a small stash of ocular pharmaceuticals you keep in a locked drawer for such occasions. One is to lower the pressure, and the other one is to quell the inflammation inside his eye that is raging like a California wildfire.

You would like to give him some pressure-lowering pills too, but it's after hours, the in-house pharmacy is closed, and nearly everyone else has gone home.

You ask where he's staying, and he gives you the name of a local homeless shelter. You tell him a social worker will come find him tomorrow and help him return to the clinic to get the pills.

He heads out the door and back to the streets. You wonder if you'll ever see him again. You think about little else that night. You're very quiet over dinner because your brain, including the parts where words and screams are formed, is fried. You sleep fretfully.

The next day, the homeless man is the first thought on your mind. You go to work and find the social worker and ask her to find the man. She locates him and makes arrangements to bring him in.

When he arrives, he says his eye feels a little better with the drops. But when you measure his vision, he says he can no longer see your hand, only light. You examine him with your slit lamp, and if anything, the cataract is even bigger and the bulging iris displaced even further forward. His intraocular pressure has risen to 52 mmHg.

You prescribe the pressure-lowering pills and make him take one before he hits the streets again. You've already called and made arrangements for him to be admitted to the ophthalmology department at your main facility for surgery. You try to explain to him how important it is that he keeps this appointment, how his eye will become even more blind and painful if he waits.

You tell him he needs to arrive early at your clinic the next morning to catch the shuttle to Birmingham and remind him that he'll probably be hospitalized for several days. He doesn't like this one bit—he's not the type of guy who likes to be pinned down and held captive to a regimented routine. You persist, though, gently at first, then more firmly.

He voices his understanding of all this and promises he will be there on time, but you know the odds are he's simply telling you what he thinks you want to hear so he can get out of there and move on. The social worker gives him city bus passes to make it easier for him. He walks out the door and back onto the streets. You wonder, once more, if you'll ever see him again.

You do all this while trying to provide quality care to the other fifteen or so regularly scheduled patients already on your plate that day.

The next morning, he doesn't show for his scheduled shuttle.

A few days later during your lunch break, you read in the online edition of your local paper about a man who was hit by a car and killed while crossing a major thoroughfare. The story names the victim, and you recognize him as your patient. The car had hit him from the right, his blind side.

On the drive home, you think about your country's health care system and your role in it. You know it's not really a "system," because that word implies a well-coordinated arrangement of smoothly moving parts.

You picture it as more of a million-piece jigsaw puzzle that has spilled onto the floor. You spend your days, some days more than others, scrambling like mad, picking up the jagged pieces and trying to assemble them into some kind of coherent, meaningful picture.

You think about the people who speak glibly of health care, who speak ill of "government doctors" like you, who dismiss the need for health care reform with the wave of a hand and opine that catch-as-catch-can ER care is "good enough" for patients like yours.

You find yourself muttering things under your breath about such people, words and phrases you thought you'd never say, ones that would disappoint and anger your mother and cause her to smack you across the mouth.

You stop yourself because you want to be a better person than that, and you try to cut them some slack.

When you arrive home, you consider the cardinal signs of professional burnout—exhaustion, cynicism, and second-guessing both your abilities and your odds of making a significant difference—and you realize you're so dangerously close to self-immolation your face is flushed and you're starting to smolder.

You reach for a ten-dollar bottle of halfway decent Cabernet to help douse the fire. You pour yourself a glass, the red line rising full to the brim. You turn toward your keyboard, and you pour out your soul.

---

**MICHAEL BROWN** is a writer, retired optometrist, and teacher who practiced for thirty years with the U.S. Department of Veterans Affairs. He received his doctorate from the University of Alabama at Birmingham and a Master of Health Science from Duke University School of Medicine. Brown has published over sixty peer-reviewed articles. He writes the Substack blog *Time Will Tell*.

POEM

# What Does a Medical Student Do All Day?

MAYA J. SORINI

I watch them while
They pull out clots
When they are gone
I clean her red

The girl goes ghost
I sternal rub
I call a code
I keep my head

I hold her up
I yield the floor
They save her life
I push the bed

I'm left alone
With just the man
I tell him that
His baby's dead.

---

**MAYA J. SORINI** is a narrative medicine scholar, medical student, essayist, and award-winning poet. Her first collection, *The Boneheap in the Lion's Den*, won the 2023 Press 53 Award for poetry and was a semifinalist for the 2024 Poetry Society of Virginia North American Book Award. She earned an MS in narrative medicine from Columbia University.

ESSAY

# D/D

## MAUREEN HIRTHLER

*My past is everything I failed to be.*

—Fernando Pessoa, *The Book of Disquiet*

AFTER YOU BROUGHT her home from the hospital, tucked her into the guest bed, and turned on the oxygen, the only magazine you could find was *Sports Illustrated*. So, lying in bed next to your mother, you are reading aloud a story about retired NBA star Charles Barkley while you watch her die. "Every Black kid thinks the only way he can be successful is through athletics. That is a terrible thing." You say *turrible thing* in your best Barkley voice, even though you know your mother wouldn't get the reference. She never understood your interest in sports; that was one of the ways in which you disappointed her. If your mother had been conscious, she would not have appreciated the irony of hearing Charles Barkley in his own words, but instead would have chosen to note you never really loved her at all.

You count the seconds between agonal breaths and know it won't be long. Your mother was proud that you were a doctor; if only you had come back to your hometown and been a family practitioner. She listed ambition among your flaws, right after being too smart and not afraid to show it. A lack of humility, she said; overreaching, thinking too highly of yourself.

Never satisfied.

*What did you do now?* Her typical response to all your failures and disappointments hovers over your head. Some of them certainly were your fault, but not all of them, even though it has taken years for you to intermittently believe that. She was a spotlight aimed directly at you, a continuous interrogation of all your decisions. You couldn't help but believe that you were responsible for every poor medical outcome, every failed relationship—you weren't intelligent enough, hadn't worked hard enough, hadn't given enough—*What did you do this time?*

*You are so uncaring. You love your father more than me. You just want me gone.* No, you just couldn't bear to watch them both suffer as every single bone of her back and chest disintegrated into an osteoporotic dust of pain. There was nothing you could do for her except let her go. The other doctors wanted to put her on a ventilator, but you knew she wouldn't recover, and if she did, the pain would be unbearable. You were the only child, the daughter, the doctor; the decisions were yours.

It is thirty seconds between breaths now; her pulse is weak and tired. The doctor knows; the daughter goes to get her father. You are on one side, him on the other. The magazine flutters to the floor. You hold her hands; the wait is short. You take out your stethoscope and listen, a full minute by the clock as you have been taught. Your father asks *How will you know?* You smile sadly. *I'm a doctor*, you say, recording the time and witnesses as you pronounce your own mother dead. Only then can you, the daughter, cry.

---

**MAUREEN HIRTHLER** is a retired physician who holds an MFA from the University of Missouri-Kansas City. Her work has appeared in *The Examined Life Journal, Pulse, Hektoen International: A Journal of Medical Humanities, JAMA*, and *Creative Nonfiction*. She lives on the coast of the Gulf of Mexico with her rescue dog, Lola, who is the queen of the palace.

POEM

# Chronic Black Excellence

MICHAEL ARNOLD

A hundred years ago, Abraham Flexner
Eulogized Black medicine.
The ink in his pen tattooed
A sleeve on the arm of systemic racism.
The idea that screamed off his report
And echoed the loudest throughout history
Was the notion that Black medicine
Was fundamentally inadequate.

For the last century, Black medicine
Has been self-medicating with Black excellence.
A treatment plan that may be just as bad
As the prevailing social illness.
Black excellence is a poisoned apple,
Being eaten by a Trojan Horse.
Side effects may include:
Elitist attitudes, reactionary logic
Burnout, brunch addiction
And respectability politics.

The siren song of Black excellence
Has veered us completely off course.
It's a self-appointed pedestal that
Makes us look down on the
People that we dreamed of healing.
It makes us want to walk away
From the neighborhoods that
Raised us and never look back.

Black excellence is a blade on
The tongue of Horatio Alger's descendants;
White people who will cut and paste
Your story into anecdotal evidence
That absolves them of their privilege.
Black excellence is a weight that actively
Compresses our humanity,
Erasing the mere possibility
Of us being normal, regular or average.
It erases the relief of mediocrity
That many of our white colleagues
Comfortably enjoy during their careers.

Who is Black excellence for exactly?
What's the message we are trying to send?
Who are we sending it to?
Are we trying to claim that we are better
Than the Black people who lifted us up

High enough to access the white-dominated
Space called Western medicine?
Are we trying to signal that we
Are one of the "good ones"?
Is it an attempt to exorcise the demons
Of ever-haunting stereotypes?
Or is it just our insecurities
Crying out, wanting desperately
For white people to finally believe
That we are adequate?

**MICHAEL ARNOLD** is a family medicine doctor affiliated with Neighborhood Family Practice in Cleveland, Ohio. He received his medical degree from Ohio University Heritage College of Osteopathic Medicine in Athens, where he was introduced to and fell in love with narrative medicine. Arnold also holds a BA from Brown University.

ESSAY

# Managed Care

JENNIFER ANDERSON

When she told me she'd walked to the bridge late that afternoon, I didn't press for details. It was not best practice for the nurse to probe. She'd already rehashed the events to the psychiatrist and therapist on admission. I don't remember if she'd planned to jump or if she'd climbed over the guardrail after replaying the events of her high school day. I do remember how she explained to me her decision to fall backward, eighteen feet to the rocks below, because she didn't want to see the ground rushing toward her face.

It was a miracle she was alive, walking around the gymnasium in the psychiatric hospital with an incomplete fracture of her cervical spine, rating her pain zero out of ten. Though she'd been cleared of a neck brace, I couldn't help but think about the cracks in her vertebrae, the vulnerability of her adolescent spine. When the football sailed lengthwise across the gym, toward the corner where she stood with her back to the ball, she neither turned nor flinched. I did. The pigskin missed her by inches before tumbling end-over-end past her feet. In a tone clipped with fear, I instructed the teenage boy to warn his peers if a wayward ball was headed their way. Especially hers, I didn't say. I softened my voice and suggested she not turn her back to a ball in play, said it would be terrible to get hit in the head. She looked at me, her countenance placid, her brown eyes bored, and said she wouldn't care if she did. She turned and followed me out of the gym.

*The Crisis Prevention Institute, equipping caregivers to recognize and safely address patients in crisis, defines rational detachment as the ability to stay in control of one's own behavior and not take the behavior of others personally.*

I don't remember how we all ended up on the floor. My coworker, one of the best in crises, shared my approach to delay going hands-on when a patient was in distress. Sometimes running down the halls and tipping chairs was sufficient release. Though this ten-year-old boy denied any history of abuse, his vigilance and reactivity said otherwise. I can't recall the inciting event that upset him. Sometimes there are few outward signs. When he began to punch his face, my coworker and I moved toward him and the three of us became entangled on the floor. I held his flailing arms. My coworker slipped his hand beneath the boy's head. He was trying to slam his skull against the linoleum, his face red and contorted in the trying, begging us to kill him, this ten-year-old boy who played with toys and still believed in magic, in superpowers, in spells.

They were getting younger and younger, these children wanting death. For the second time in two decades as a nurse, I failed to restrain my tears.

I don't remember how long he took to calm, when all that self-hatred and rage slithered off to wait and hide, how much he was willing to debrief or not. I do remember that we offered him something to eat and drink, engaged him in conversation about his favorite Power Rangers character, then printed more coloring sheets before walking him back to group. I apologized to my coworker about failing to remain detached. He removed his glasses and wiped his eyes.

*According to the Attachment, Regulation, Competency (ARC) Framework, Caregiver Affect Management involves a foundational building block of attachment wherein the caregiver recognizes and regulates her own emotional and physiological experience so she can then attune to and support those in her care.*

The fifteen-year-old girl was medically stable; a voluntary, though reluctant, admission to the psychiatry unit. It was the time of year when the days were filled with more darkness than light, sometime in the hours between dinner and bed. Not that she'd eaten much since the doctors pumped from her stomach what they could of her mother's painkillers. You'd think hospice would have removed them from the house.

One rectangular table and five chairs crowded the small interview room. She sat down in the furthest seat and crossed her arms. Her tall father had the good looks of waning youth—tan, lean, muscled, strong. His baseball hat shadowed his eyes, narrowed and darkened, as if they'd already seen too much. They had. He'd watched his wife, the one in the ground, deteriorate in a matter of months. They'd been together two-thirds of their lives.

The younger brother shared his father's likeness, though none of his anger, which lurked, quiet, in the cage of his body. The boy sat patiently, hands tucked under his legs, fixing his eyes on the table, the safest spot to look. I explained the stack of legal paperwork before passing the papers first to the daughter. She signed them in haste before shoving them toward her father, her eyes daring him to look at her while he scribbled his name. He wouldn't. I described the estimated length of stay, daily schedules, the roles of the interdisciplinary team who would prescribe medications, lead group therapy, facilitate a family meeting, create a safety plan. No one had comments or questions. Grief was the loudest, largest presence in the room.

After her family left, it was just her and me in the interview room. There were questions nurses asked only after a parent or guardian had gone. I typed her responses into the computer, assessing her levels of anxiety, depression, hopelessness, safety, watching and listening for cues about when she wanted to elaborate and when she didn't. She talked about how she stopped having people over to her house, that nearly every night her father came home drunk and bloody from the fights he'd start at the bar. His mother had recently moved in to help. Some nights he'd stay with his girlfriend, a nurse in another town. The father who fights, the daughter in flight, the son who freezes. I typed, pausing to wipe the tears from my face, unable, for the first time in all my years as a nurse, to keep my feelings inside.

After finishing the admission and hospital tour, I brought her belongings to her room. A photo stuck out from between the pages of her book. She pulled it out and showed me. Her mom had kind eyes, a pretty smile. I told her that I imagined her mom's absence was like a fire that went out, pulling the warmth and light from every room. Her eyes met mine. Yes.

It was near midnight when I left the hospital. I was grateful for my thirty-minute commute. When a song came on the radio about a man who says he's fine when he's not, about the empty place at the table where she used to sit, about how he only sees her when he dreams, I cried the whole way home.

*Distress Tolerance, one of Dialectical Behavioral Therapy's four skill modules, involves Crisis Survival Skills to move through instead of worsen distress, and Reality Acceptance Skills to prevent suffering and increase personal control.*

His was the first patient's wake I'd ever attended. I wish it were my last. He was admitted to the hospital after he cut the phone line when his family left the house, then started the engine in the garage. His mom returned home to pick up something she'd forgotten.

He loved four-wheeling, hunting, dirt bikes, and sugar. Winsome, foul-mouthed, handsome, hilarious. Sixteen. I still remember his room safety check. He'd managed to flatten half a dozen soda cans so they were hidden behind the BMX posters he had taped to the walls. When I loosened the paper from the ceiling, candy wrappers rained down all over his bed. I laughed. He was the reason the hospital would later ban posters in patients' rooms. I asked him why he'd hidden all the wrappers—the aluminum cans, considered contraband, I understood. He told me he'd read in the teen handbook (he'd been bored) that he wasn't supposed to have candy on the unit, somehow it had slipped by staff, and so he hid the evidence to keep from getting in trouble.

Not that he avoided trouble, in or out of the hospital. Drinking, skipping school, fighting with his father. He lingered in the halls, resisted going to bed, needed frequent reminders not to swear. I found it hard to redirect him with any seriousness because his humor was so disarming. A great way to deflect and avoid. I learned from him, and would have years to practice, that there is an art to addressing behavior, that all behavior communicates something, that some images will stay with you always. Like the BMX posters and his easy grin, the candy wrappers scattered across his narrow hospital bed, his open-mouthed coffin, the tie and starched collar pulled high and tight to hide his neck.

*Joyce University of Nursing and Health Sciences identifies the four stages of compassion fatigue, often experienced by caregivers regularly exposed to significant stress and trauma, as the Zealot Phase, the Irritability Phase, the Withdrawal Phase, and the Zombie Phase; suggested antidote: improved self-care.*

---

**JENNIFER ANDERSON** worked for twenty-three years as an inpatient psychiatric nurse for children and adolescents. She holds an MFA in creative nonfiction from Antioch University and is enrolled in the Narrative Medicine Certification of Professional Achievement program at Columbia University. Her essays have appeared in *The Missouri Review* and *Iron Horse Literary Review*. She lives in Wisconsin with her husband and their three teens.

# 4
# LOST IN TRANSLATION

*Confusion*

ESSAY

# Ambulance Stories

## B. SHEPARD BLUE

I TOOK A young boy to the hospital with a broken arm after he fell off his trampoline. As I took vital signs, my partner asked him how he fell; how high; what hurt; how much it hurt; if he could feel the touch of gloved fingers, squeeze my partner's hand; if he could hold this end of the splint while I bound it to his forearm with gauze. He was stone-faced and stoic, and I was annoyed with him at first. His bare-bones acknowledgment of our presence, eyes focused anywhere but our faces, made him stiff when I asked him to move or asked a question.

Then I heard the choke in his voice and saw how he was fighting not to cry in front of the keen eyes of his mother, perched nearby and watching. From one man to another, I understood.

The watchful eyes of his mother—I noticed she hadn't spoken a word. I kept glancing at her, awaiting something, anything from her. I cast a small, unsympathetic judgment onto her and her distance from us.

Then the boy explained his mother was deaf. I almost laughed; then I picked up my hands and began to sign, dredging up my memories of American Sign Language. I saw the relief in his mother's keen eyes as communication opened. The questions I had been waiting for came in force. Suddenly everything felt complete: a boy with a broken arm, an EMT, and now the watching mother.

His mother rode in the back of the ambulance with us. I signed as I spoke to the boy, allowing her to be part of our conversation—to eavesdrop in her own way, as mothers need to. My sign language was slow and deliberate, unpracticed compared to her beautifully fluid signs, but thankfully comprehensible.

Afterward, I began to wonder. I rewound the encounter back and forth in my head. I wondered why the boy didn't sign with his mother. His unbroken arm stayed in his lap the entire time; his mother's only view into his words were the movements of his lips. I wondered about the separation between them. Having an intermediary to communicate seemed too routine to them. I also wondered about the disconnect between her and the world—with no small amount of shame on my initial prejudice. Just some of those small questions that bubble up in hindsight as I rewind the memory over and over.

---

I took an old man home from a hospital after he fell and hit his head. A label in his patient record rattled in all caps: FIGHT RISK. It was a rare warning and a bogeyman to us. On our initial contact my partner and I stayed back, trying not to aggravate him, as if he would snap his toothless jaws at us if we got too close.

No snap ever came. I joined him in the ambulance, and we had the most pleasant conversation. We talked baseball and hockey. He had dementia and I could hear it in the winding path his words took and the thick-tongued, unsteady mumble that slurred the consonants together. His replies were often tangential to the arc of conversation, kissing its surface, then meandering in some other direction. It would be cruel to judge him for those meanderings.

Dementia dissolves the brain and its tongue like brine on limestone, turning it all into pumice. I understood him; after all, there is more to language than syntax. There is tone and word choice, facial expressions, the light in the eyes. He gave me enough clues I could understand.

After we helped him into bed, I stepped outside the room and dodged the spearheaded gazes of the onlooking caregivers. One started telling the story of the FIGHT RISK label, unprompted. "Two of us were helping him to the bathroom. He seemed normal, then he started swinging." A hand wave in his direction. "He has no idea what's going on. We were just getting him to the bathroom. God. I'm not glad he's back." No attempt to lower their voices, even with the subject within earshot and watching.

I looked at him as he sat on his bed. It's not often I see people in the early stages of dementia. Most dementia patients I take are in the late stages, gray matter dribbling out the back of their skulls as the cortex aggregates and dissolves. I saw the old man still there, though. I saw it in his eyes. My mouth stayed closed. I feel like I failed him.

I wondered how it felt to have dementia ravaging your mind, feeling the creep of fingers against the most precious, inner surface of you, skimming nails over gray matter and leaving lines in the chalkboard there, brushing away fragile, dusty writings. The image was vivid to me as I looked at him sitting there, diapered, shriveled, hunched, glassy-eyed.

The narrative on my patient care report was dry, generic. Not writing the rest down, not transcribing it and trying to give words to something beyond language, deepened my sense of failure.

I took a man home from a hospital after his tracheostomy tube was replaced. A car accident paralyzed him from the neck down and he communicated in clicks, like how you urge on a horse: one for Yes, two for No. His hands were frozen in just the right hooked shape to pull out his tracheostomy tube and land himself in the ER with a botched suicide attempt. I stood at his bedside and he looked at me. I felt uncomfortable. He had enough control over his jaw and enough mobility in his shattered skull plates that he could make a grotesque noise by grinding them together with a chewing motion. He saw my discomfort and he made the grinding noise all the way home. I didn't blame him for extracting schadenfreude from the latex-gloved hands of medicine that pinned him here. After transferring him from the stretcher to his cot, the flat-eyed caregiver assumed responsibility from me and I ducked out, feeling those eyes, those human eyes, those eyes with no language against my back. I still hear his sounds. He was bilingual, in a way: his prosthetic language made of Yes and No, and the indecipherable language of his own creation, the grinding of his skull. A hopelessly binary language: Yes and No. How do you condense a being into Yes and No? You don't; you supplement your Yes and No with grinding: metallic, harsh—angry, despairing. The grinding language of his own creation—unique to him and his nightmare—worked better to communicate than any other language.

—

My coworker almost took someone to the hospital.

He kept the story short. "I had someone die on the rig today."

"That sucks." I kept it short too.

"Yeah."

"I'm sorry."

What else is there to say? We left spaces between the words—huge, immense spaces—trying to make room for the colossus of death. The back of an ambulance is barely big enough for both a ghost and an EMT. In such a tight space, you feel compelled to ration your words. A single person is so immense.

—

I took a man to a mental health hospital.

As told by the nurse, he came in for suicidal ideation after the death of a roommate sent him into a spiral. The section listing the bullet-point diagnoses of his medical history, titled a "problem list," told a sad, lonely story: depression, anxiety, alcoholism, and high risk of homosexual behavior.

I will never forget those words. What a diagnosis! "High risk" listed under the patient's "problem list"; a man on the brink of suicide; God save him, he loved another man.

I wondered if I were standing in 1980.

I gathered my iPad off the Formica countertop. The beige-speckled linoleum, reminiscent of a school cafeteria, was lined with off-blue plastic molding dusted with hair and dirt. It all felt unclean and dated.

Hindsight is a demon and our long drive left her plenty of time to work. That was not a roommate who died, but how else would he describe the man he lived with to medicine? The medicine that would affix the pink triangle of "high risk of homosexual behavior" to him, on the same level as the depression and anxiety that led him to peer over the edge of a bridge at night? The same medicine that would, after such a crippling loss and a mislabeling of "roommate," shunt him on an ambulance ride forty-five minutes away?

He said he didn't bring his glasses to the emergency room with him. He said the streetlamps looked like Christmas lights to him in the blurriness. I said, "I know what you mean," and I took my glasses off and set them on the bench beside me. We sat looking at the lights together, bleary and blotted with the early, watery morning, watching the will-o'-the-wisps wandering away in the darkness.

After transferring care, I climbed into the ambulance and shut the door. I looked over my shoulder, back at the hospital. I saw him through a window watching the ambulance. I doubted he could see inside the dark cab but, with the bright lights in the hospital, I could see him. He nodded at the cab. The same nod you give a stranger in respectful acknowledgment, a brief connection between two people who will never see each other again. He looked resolute, enduring.

I think he'll be all right, despite everything.

I took a young boy to the emergency room from a group home. His insurance read one name and his nurse stated another. His sex marker was a graceless, ambiguous T. I recognized the story being told to me—after all, it was my story as well. These idiosyncrasies were the awkward attempts of medicine to collapse the transgender experience into a medical record. I understood.

The nurse quipped that he'd say he doesn't speak English when, really, he does. I smiled at the eye roll in her voice. I remembered the flippant anger of adolescence, purposeless save for thin satisfaction.

A young boy emerged moodily from a darkened room, the hood of his sweater pulled over his head. He sat himself silently on the gurney and shut his eyes during our assessment, defying the situation by feigning sleep.

While on the rig, I commented on a section of beads strung in his hair: blue then pink then white, then pink and blue again. The colors of our pride flag. I mentioned I was transgender too. "Really?" he said—those eyes opened fast—and suddenly he could speak perfect, fluent English. He talked the whole way to the hospital.

He said he didn't like the hospital we were taking him to because it made him "uncomfortable." Sometimes he'd say he didn't speak English when, really, he can.

I asked what happens when they bring out the Spanish interpreter. "I say I don't speak Spanish."

I believed he would be in and out of the ER for an open-and-shut case of strep. When we arrived at the hospital, I was expecting to sign off and quietly leave with a "Good night" and well wishes. Then his nurse, in accordance with a bizarre policy, asked him to remove all his clothes and wear a gown.

His tears bubbled up instantly and I saw that word "uncomfortable" appear, wrenching, and I interpreted it as gender dysphoria. Both as a caregiver and as another transgender man, I did my best to advocate for him.

I fought quietly, politely with the nurse, but policy and one-size-fits-all bureaucracy won. I had to tell the boy I tried but didn't succeed. His voice tightened again, and he cried. I watched and I wondered. Was this something else? I couldn't shake it. The sudden shyness. The tears. The body, exposure.

I asked if something else was going on. I looked at him, leaning weight into the "something else" to convey what I actually meant. I knew he understood; he was old enough to.

"No," he said through tears.

"Do you feel safe at home?"

The casual language and rapport I built with him dried up and fell from my dialogue. I leaned into scripted phrases I vaguely remembered from work trainings.

"Yes," he replied, shakily.

I said, "Okay." I took a breath then said, "I'm a mandated reporter. If I feel like something is going on, or you tell me something is going on, I have to tell someone." We kept referring to it as something, not naming the topic at hand but aware of it.

"Yeah."

"Did something else happen at home?" I asked again. I couldn't say, "Did somebody touch you?" It felt too visceral for me to say as I felt memories return.

"Yeah."

I felt the rest of the planet being swallowed by a black hole, leaving us alone in space. I looked at the crying boy before me and froze. I clung to standard, scripted phrases, and gathered the information I could. The thin connection of trust in our shared transgender experience barely kept the doors of conversation open. Even with the vagaries and euphemisms on my part and half-mumbled, shameful affirmatives from him, I knew we were referring to the same something that happened.

I left quietly and informed the nurse, who said, "Okay."

I had never filled out a child abuse report form in my life. The "clinicality" of it was both jarring and a relief. I hope I never fill out another. I felt like the earth was shaking under me the entire time. I couldn't escape the reminder of my own long-gone childhood. I heard and felt those echoes. The physical feeling of it. It never goes away. The ghost of hands. They creep under the skin and leave imprints on the soft tissue of your nerves like handprints in wet concrete, and when those nerves fire again you feel the phantom limbs, the divots in the shape of palms, fingers.

In his pain I saw parallels in mine. "Don't touch me; don't look at me," he was saying with his body language and discomfort with the hospital gown. I knew. I understood.

---

**B. SHEPARD BLUE** is a former paramedic, now nearing graduation from medical school in California. His years working on an ambulance inform his careers in both writing and medicine and have shaped the lens through which he now approaches emergency medicine.

# The Spaces Between

JENNIFER LI

Every morning, I watch
the sun ascending through the windows—
deep, delicate quiet that fills my throat before
I clear the cobwebs out of my sinuses with
*good mornings* and dark coffee.

This morning, she is a patient with
the cadence of '60s *telenovelas*, consonants
tumbling over the cusp of psychosis—she is,
they say, both sweet and frightful, a
lesson in contradiction. She trembles, limbs
twisted and askew. *Linda*, she calls me,
"pretty" in her native tongue, pinning me down with
her gaze as if I am the early bird perched
on her windowsill. I cannot tell,
with her, if it is a compliment. Her hands
gesture at me, gnarled and shaky,
¿*hablas español? ¿me entiendes?*

The attending physician beside me is
serene, patient, aged spots lining his face
in a pattern that resembles my late grandfather,
crouched over his crinkled Chinese pathology books
laid out across his large glass desk.

"The diaspora," the attending remarks.
I feel the word sit itself inside me as viscerally
as the tug of her skin when I move
to examine her joints. She pauses, for a
brief, clear moment. *Sí*, she says.
It is the shortest phrase she has spoken amongst
the tumbling of syllables fighting to be heard—

Her thoughts, like a diaspora,
remain scattered. Scattered brain, localized
damage, a scattered, localized population.
Displaced, scarred, darkened
velvety skin over her unnaturally curved spine.
When I let go of her hands,
she flings them out once more.
*Estoy muriendo*, she announces, over and over—
"I am dying"—and her daughter beside her
sighs, a barely-there huff of breath into the stale air.

"As are we all," the attending responds,
in English, calm and thoughtful.

Outside, in the hall, someone laughs.
When my grandfather died,
I watched reruns of slapstick cartoons on mute,
fingers numb around his leftover calligraphy brushes,
steeped myself in raw, unbridled silence until
I finally looked up *congestive heart failure* and learned
to scrape the pain out of the hollow of my throat.

*Estoy muriendo*, she moans again,
louder. Her daughter is writing in a notebook.
I am the only one listening. I reach for
her legs to feel for swelling.
I try, fruitlessly, to smooth out the
wrinkles in the fabric of her pant legs.
She is abruptly silent.

When I look up, she is smiling,
like she has been waiting for this moment,
her smile merely momentarily misplaced,
lost in the dispersion. *Linda*, she tells me again.
Her legs are still, and I roll her ankle
into the spaces between my fingers.

In the quiet, the attending begins
to type. A ray of sun unfolds from
the open window. I can still taste the remnants

of coffee in the corners of my mouth.

*Entiendo. Gracias.*

*Thank you*

---

**JENNIFER LI** is an academic hospitalist at Grady Memorial Hospital in Atlanta. She graduated with a BA in English literature and an MD from Emory University. In medical school, she was an editor for *in-Training* and on an advisory board focused on diversity called *Mosaic in Medicine*; she is now a nonfiction editor for *Intima*. She enjoys playing piano and tennis, attending indie concerts, and watching art films.

ESSAY

# When Suicide Speaks Arabic

IBRAHIM SABLABAN

BEING THE SON of Arab refugees can grant you a unique perspective. One I don't think many people understand—or *can* understand. Secrecy, the ever-present air of fear and insularity, were all hallmarks of my upbringing. For better or worse, I always felt like an alien. It all still seems completely reasonable to me, and I say that being a psychiatrist. My experiences had their handicaps, but as life unfolded, I found them to be of far more utility than I would have ever imagined.

I was working in a consultation service back in residency at the hospital where I trained.

We got called on for mental health–related admissions, from psychoses to suicides. My colleagues and I were consulted on the case of a Syrian boy in his teens, Rafiq. He and his family were refugees from the Middle East who had ultimately ended up being resettled in the United States. He hadn't experienced the trauma of war directly, but he and his family had lost everything in their displacement and moved several times before getting here. Along the way, through the turmoil, he met a girl he'd sparked with. But his resettlement caused their long-distance relationship to founder and die. The day after they broke up, he was admitted for a suicide attempt. He was caught by his family overdosing on a bottle of pain medication.

Although I was the one who reviewed the chart, a white

colleague of mine was assigned to the case. He emerged from Rafiq's room about thirty minutes later with fairly encouraging news.

"His attempt was impulsive and out of character. The bottle wasn't full, and this kid's got aspirations . . . he's got family. His father's supportive and on board. I don't think he's in danger. The attempt was haphazard, more a cry for help."

According to my colleague, Rafiq acted impulsively. Having a girlfriend and not marrying her was a big deal in the culture, but Rafiq felt as though he'd overreacted in the aftermath of the breakup. His father would be there to support him through his emotional trauma and was willing to do whatever it took to help. Besides, Rafiq and his family were devout Muslims. In the literature, religious affiliation is a massive protective factor against suicide.

And so our team developed a plan. We'd send young Rafiq home, enroll him in a structured treatment program, and get him close outpatient follow-up afterward. He and his father were in agreement. This was, of course, all voluntary and unmonitored. But still reasonable. In fact, we got cases like that almost every day. Teenage love leads to impulsivity, known the world over.

But something didn't *feel* right.

This wasn't just another patient. He was a refugee. His dad was a refugee. As a Muslim, an Arab, and the son of displaced parents myself, I couldn't wrap my head around how smoothly everything had gone. As haphazard as this suicide attempt (which we'd all but stopped calling it) was, I couldn't imagine devout Muslim Arabs from abroad taking it so *well*. Suicide is a massive deal in the Islamic faith, the dishonor of it is arguably a bigger deal in Arab culture.

I had to see him for myself.

I walked by Rafiq's room, peeking in, and the face he wore betrayed the story we'd just heard. He was looking up at the ceiling, jaw clenched, eyes red and tears streaming down his cheeks.

His face looked paralyzed with anger and he was utterly silent as I approached. I saw the father sitting as far away from his son's bed as he could, with a blank gaze off into nowhere. There was a coldness between them. A feeling of dread permeated the room. I walked in and introduced myself. They both turned to me and composed themselves, immediately forcing smiles. *Assalamualaikum*, I said: "Peace be upon you," in Arabic. Again, a change in affect—a startled confusion. They responded, *Waalaikumsalam*: "Peace upon you as well."

I decided to speak exclusively in Arabic to Rafiq and his father. I had to. I had already heard their story in English, and from my experience, it could be a distant language. Spoken without much emotion. Easy to twist narratives and lose meanings in. But Arabic was their mother tongue. Our mother tongue. I asked Rafiq's father to leave the room so I could speak to his son privately.

The facade didn't last long. Rafiq recounted his story, and after a few minutes started talking at length, tears in his eyes. He told me he was morbidly depressed. About how he started failing classes as his relationship crumbled. How he had lost weight. How he couldn't bring himself to get up in the morning. How he wanted to go home and be left alone. We pause and take a moment.

"Your father didn't look too happy," I say.

He chuckles. "Would yours be?"

The topic shifted away from his lost love, and to him. "I'm ashamed of myself. I can't believe what I've done," he went on. "I've disgraced my family and my faith. I'm cursed. I'm weak." He was speaking about himself with an air of anger.

"Do you want to kill yourself?"

"No," he meekly replied.

"Why not?"

He was silent. He struggled to give a reason, and then stopped trying. When I asked about Islam, he agreed about the sinfulness of suicide, but in a manner that didn't move him. He didn't care. This was a young man who was deeply depressed, and now, consumed by guilt. He was a tragedy waiting to happen.

Separately, I spoke to his father. He again belittled the situation, and pleaded with me that they go home, until I confronted him about the gravity of a suicide in the Islamic faith. A truly somber mood fell upon us both.

"It's apostasy." His affect changed to sadness. To disappointment. To anger. "He's ungrateful. I've sent him to school. Provided for him. I expected nothing in return. And for what? He betrayed our honor and betrayed God. Had he died, he would have gone to hell. He can't be my son."

The father went on. His idea of treatment was different from ours. He'd take away his son's bedroom. He'd treat him more sternly. No therapy, no follow-up, no treatment programs, no medications. He was to be punished. The father told me he didn't believe in the Americans, or their system. At the end of his rant, overcome with emotion, he cried.

This picture, I understood.

I pleaded with him in Arabic. I had to. I couldn't be the stoic Western psychiatrist I'd learned to be. Rafiq's outlook on life was entwined with his father's perception of him. I reminded him of what a blessing it was that his son didn't perish. That fate brought them to the hospital that day. To us. I had to emphasize my own religious background, and the perils my parents faced coming to the US. I quoted the Quran. To let him know that I understood. He may have been in an alien land, but at the very least, I wasn't an alien. And as we spoke, he grew more open and concerned about my perception of him and his son. Concerned with honor. A fixture of Arab culture.

Ultimately, it wasn't a Western interview technique that won the day. Not Beck or Freud either. I ended up citing *Majnun Layla* (literally "Layla's Madman"), a seventh-century Arabian tale of romance; it is the equivalent of *Romeo and Juliet* in the Middle East. The story ends with a young man driven to madness and death, with pages filled with notions of dishonor and regret.

Fitting for an Arab father speaking to a psychiatrist. Far closer to Syria in spirit than to America.

And he gave me a smile. A genuine one. I was able to show him we weren't dealing with some bizarre Western perversion but a theme ever-present within our own culture as well. And that's where we started breaking down the barriers between us and treatment. Because in this case, I needed Rafiq's father to be on board to treat Rafiq effectively. I was not oblivious to the challenges they'd still face, but this would be an opportunity to facilitate better treatment. And it ultimately did.

It's probably easy to look at the story and think of the culture as a whole—Arab or Muslim culture—as inconducive to mental health. Plenty of medieval Muslim physicians and psychologists would disagree. The real problem is that refugees and immigrants are told constantly that they're *the other* and are expected not to be when they step into a hospital. The rhetoric about them externalizes them to American society. Why would they trust us with their most intimate, socially interwoven problems? My family certainly wouldn't. So as positive as this patient encounter ultimately was, I can't help but feel that it was more a story about failure than success.

---

**IBRAHIM SABLABAN** is a dual board-certified psychiatrist and addiction medicine physician in the Metro Detroit area. He is the director of medical education at Beaumont Behavioral Health and sits on the National Board of Directors for American Muslim Health Professionals, a not-for-profit public advocacy group focusing on civic and health care collaboration. The son of Palestinian refugees, Sablaban has focused on minority mental health, acculturation, and health care disparities across American urban centers.

ESSAY

# Across the Great Rift

SOPHIA GAUTHIER

"No, no." Wycliffe gently shakes his head. "*Ana*-kohoa, not *una*-kohoa."

He taps the side of his coffee mug with his pen and little ripples appear on the surface. Wycliffe and I are sitting at a wooden table outside under a white plastic tent. The morning is bright and brisk and I burrow into my fleece, frowning at my cheat sheet. My half-eaten plate of scrambled eggs is pushed off to the side and his coffee has long stopped steaming.

"Tena," he says, which means *again* in Swahili.

Five years ago, I might have been intimidated by this experience—I was intimidated by a lot of experiences, specifically those that might end in failure. But today, over eight thousand miles from home and almost seven thousand feet above sea level, I'm taking Swahili lessons in the mornings before rounding on the pediatric ward of Moi University's children's hospital in Eldoret, Kenya. It's my first time in Africa.

Wycliffe is a fantastic teacher. He is very silly and when he laughs, he bounces up and down in his chair. He laughs easily.

Today, we have named his coffee mug "Wycliffe Junior." Wycliffe Junior is five years old and has a chest cold. I am supposed to be taking Wycliffe Junior's medical history, but I keep asking, "Are *you* coughing?" instead of looking at Wycliffe and asking, "Is *he* coughing?"

Wycliffe believes that I am having difficulty with conjugation. To be fair, I usually am having difficulty with conjugation, but I don't know how to explain to him that in the US we often ask children directly about their symptoms. "How are you feeling?" "Does your throat hurt today?" The culture shift is subtle, but it's one of the first things I notice about practicing medicine in Kenya. The hierarchy is stricter here. At a speaker presentation a few nights ago, a Kenyan man held his hand horizontally in front of his forehead. He said, "Here is God." He lowered his hand a half an inch and said, "Here are doctors."

Wycliffe nods toward my eggs.

"Please, eat!" and he relaxes in his chair, indicating that we don't need to rush the lesson.

He can tell that I am unaccustomed to the leisurely pace and smiles wistfully.

―

Rachel tugs gently at the elbow of my white coat. She is quiet and nervous, speaks like she is humming, and I cannot hear her. I tilt my head.

She swallows and tries again, unconsciously pressing her fingers to the hearing aid in her right ear, like it will help me hear her better too.

"Can you tell me why Kamau's left arm is so . . . puffy?" I tilt my head in confusion. I haven't examined Kamau. I haven't examined most of our patients today. I spent the majority of rounds scrolling through the medical database UpToDate, trying to remember the primary metastatic spread of a Wilms's tumor. I color at my mental absence.

Rachel is a fourth-year Kenyan medical student and I am an American pediatric fellow. We are rounding on the same pediatric hospital medicine team. As a foreign visitor, I'm still figuring out how to be an asset here.

We make our way together across the ward. It is a small room, but the journey takes time.

We weave clumsily through a sea of family members, some cradling purple plastic dishes of ugali and beans, some carting young babies wrapped to their backs in kitenge slings, some driving small children to their beds, a firm palm on the back of their heads. My white coat catches on a bed frame; I bump into a nurse.

Most of the beds cradle two patients, their sleepy parents, their neatly stacked possessions. They watch us on rounds, us and our unwieldy white coats, us fiddling with notecards, us exchanging portable pulse oximeters, us flipping through pink patient folders, us fumbling with the shoestrings that secure our medical notes.

Us shaking our heads.

Many families only speak the local dialects of their ancestors. Our Big, Important Medical Discussions are in capital "E" English, and they nod and smile when we use words like "leukemia" and "encephalopathy" to describe their children.

Rachel and I finally land in the corner of the room. Kamau is sitting up, his eyes are big and curious and yellow like an owl, his front teeth gently gnawing on his bottom lip. I kneel in front of Kamau and his mother.

I introduce myself in rudimentary Swahili and they nod politely. I unzip Kamau's sweatshirt. It is dirty, speckled with old blood after a failed IV. Kamau is six years old but cannot weigh more than fifteen kilos—less than thirty-five pounds. He has a stippled mass the size of a grapefruit fixed to the left side of his neck. The otolaryngologists have been hesitant to biopsy it because he has not been able to maintain a hemoglobin level above seven. Blood is scarce.

Rachel points to his arms, and I take his wrists and extend them into the light. His skin stretches taut over his bones, like a sheepskin drying in the sun. I am gentle as I rotate his wrist, because I feel like there can't possibly be enough muscle to hold his joints in place.

Kamau's left forearm is disproportionately plump. I press my thumb into the belly of his wrist, and when I remove it, there is a soft impression. I ask Rachel to run her hands over the mark.

"Pitting edema," she says. She looks back at me, a question poised on her lips. I wonder if Kamau's neck mass is starting to compress his subclavian vein.

While I am talking to Rachel, I forget that I am still holding Kamau's left wrist. I feel a soft tug at the back of my neck and notice that Kamau has reached out with his free hand and is examining the bell of my stethoscope. I laugh involuntarily. He is so weak and so small, but in that moment, he fills my entire space. I can no longer hear the moans from bed seventeen, or the screams from the procedure room.

Rachel and I need to rejoin rounds. I close my fingers around his tiny hand and squeeze.

It is warm and still full of life. "Goodbye, Kamau," and I let go.

―

The death book is a black-and-white marble composition notebook. This one is well used: It has masking tape on the binding and its pages are thick and crinkled with ink. It sits against the wall in the corner of the nurses' station, under the admission book and a stack of lab requisition forms.

It took me a while to find the death book. I didn't know how to ask for it. Imagine me and my thick American accent flippantly asking around for a "death book," because it's obvious that I trained in a part of the world where we don't have a need for one. I don't know if the local staff even call it the death book. But other visiting trainees do, and they whisper about it like the world's worst-kept secret, so I went looking.

I leaf through the pages; there are hundreds of entries from this year alone. Each page is dedicated to a single patient, like a headstone. The first paragraph is a summary of their hospital stay. It reads professionally: "four-year-old male with lymphoma" or "nine-year-old female with difficulty breathing . . ." The second paragraph is a summary of the events leading up to their death. Kamau's entry reads, "at 12:32 AM, child found with pupils fixed and dilated."

I've only been at the hospital for two weeks but I know three of the patients listed.

Here in Eldoret, death on the pediatric wards is routine. I've been told that one in eight children who walk through the hospital doors leave by way of the mortuary. To be clear, the patient population here is sicker and the access to intensive monitoring is limited. These are children who come from all over, tribes in Kenya's interior, even Tanzania, Uganda, Sudan. They make the expensive journey because they can no longer afford to delay care.

In a few short weeks, I have become accustomed to death; I have forgotten that we are allowed to grieve. When a young mother is screaming and pounding her fists into the concrete floor, crying out for her child as staff wrap him in a shroud and cart him away, we have to turn our backs and move on to the next patient.

However, the death book tells a different story. Every entry ends with "RIP." It feels powerfully sentimental for the sterility of a medical record, a testament that the staff here are mourning too, ensuring the memories of their patients are stamped in permanent ink.

---

The Maasai Mara is a nationally protected game reserve in western Kenya, contiguous with the Serengeti in neighboring Tanzania.

It's noontime, the equatorial sun blazing overhead, and an impala struggles to give birth. She is naked and vulnerable in the savannah, nothing but wispy grasses to offer cover for miles. Finally, her calf spills unceremoniously onto the earth. It is uncoordinated and covered in blood and stringy amniotic fluid. It writhes in the dirt below the shade of its mother's loose belly. The two are exhausted.

Within an hour after the birth, two male lions are panting under the same unrelenting sun. One is sitting on the ground, guarding the mother impala, dead and bloody at his side. The other is trotting away, the broken neck of the calf clenched in his jaws, its scrawny legs swinging, hooves scaping the soil.

A violent birth transitions into a violent death and all I can think about are the inevitabilities of place. Back in an American children's hospital, we like to call our patients resilient. They *are* resilient. But it strikes me that they are also lucky.

In contrast, here in sub-Saharan Africa, at a facility where family members line up to donate blood because there isn't enough in stock, in a hospital where patients with cancer share beds with patients with tuberculosis because there simply is no space, in a country where about one third of the population lives on less than two dollars a day, I see Kamau in my dreams, I beg for forgiveness, I grieve for his mourning mother, and I think about the rotten *luck* of his loss.

―

On my last day in Kenya, we hike a steep dirt path through the Kerio Valley to the base of Torok Falls. It is an impressive 150-meter column of cold water. It cascades from the top of a towering escarpment 2,400 meters above sea level, home to some of the greatest running champions the world has ever seen.

I am winded and poorly acclimated to the altitude, but this is the daily school path for many of the local children who live on the surrounding farmland. They call out to us and giggle when we wave back. At one point, we pass a young boy hauling a wooden table down the mountain to sell at market. It's hoisted over his left shoulder, and he deftly descends past our hiking boots in a pair of leather sandals.

Our tour guide beams with pride when he tells me that his sixteen-year-old daughter finished second in the regional cross-country meet. He's been hiking this route for twenty years and barely breaks a sweat. He's met tourists from all over the world, faraway places I've never heard of, but he himself has never set foot outside of Kenya.

When we reach the base of the waterfall we are drenched by icy waves of spray, and I scream into the valley because I feel so wonderfully alive. My voice dissipates into the rift. To our guide, the Kerio Valley is not some novel tourist attraction; it is home. He knows how cold the water gets, so he keeps dry at a careful distance, leaning gracefully along a wind-carved tree.

---

**SOPHIA GAUTHIER** is an assistant professor of pediatrics at Duke University School of Medicine. She is a pediatric hospitalist and a storyteller with special interests in narrative medicine and global health. Her essay "Myrtle Beach" appeared in *Pulse*.

ESSAY

# It's Not That

KATHERINE FLORES GUZMAN

The patient sits across from me. She comes for weekly injections. I go over the usual education points and review her care plan. Eat healthy, get enough exercise, etc. But something seems off today. She's quieter than usual.

"What kinds of exercise have you been doing?" I ask. She lets out a sad smile.

"I'm sorry. I know what you're gonna say. I haven't been doing much exercise, actually. It's really hard to go outside nowadays."

I try to instill a little optimism. After all, part of the job is encouraging patients. "Ah, but we're expecting some good sunny days soon! It'll be easier to go outside in the nice weather, right?"

She looks down and sighs.

"No, it's not that. Every time I go outside, there is this group of gang members that stare at me and give me bad vibes. It's like they're watching me. One time, one of them followed me to my floor. They tend to stand outside my apartment building. We're planning on moving, but I just don't feel comfortable leaving my apartment when my boyfriend's not there."

I give myself a mental slap for rushing to judgment. I am reminded that I should choose my words better because sometimes our patients have a hard time with treatment compliance due to several socioeconomic factors.

"You probably don't know the area, but it's the apartments

over there around the corner." She points behind me, signaling out the window. She says it in a way that means everybody should know to stay away from there.

Sometimes I find it funny how my patients assume I won't know where they're coming from. Because in that moment, I understand her immediately. I know exactly where she is talking about. I know exactly why she is saying that, because I too grew up there. And eleven years later, the gang violence is still there, even worse. I look at this teenage mother in front of me and I see so much of myself in her.

Nevertheless, I say, "Huh. I'm not familiar with that neighborhood."

It hits too close to home. It brings back too many unwanted flashbacks. And I have to move on to the next patient.

---

**KATHERINE FLORES GUZMAN** is a nurse practitioner and writer with special interests in underserved communities and public health research. She believes in the power of language to foster empathy, create healing spaces, and honor the communities that shape us. Her writing has appeared in *Calendula Review*, *Auxocardia*, and *Yellow Arrow Journal*.

ESSAY

# Vicious

TIM CUNNINGHAM

ABDUL'S BELLY WAS swollen like the rice fields. It didn't take much rain to saturate them, the swaths of troughs and ridges, muddy dams and canals near our clinic. Hundreds and thousands of pounds of rice they produced. The growth endless, always water, always mud. Runoff lubricated the road that bifurcated the camp where we worked. From the deforested hills above where a reported eight hundred thousand Rohingyas live, torrents of water and mud carved new paths toward the fields. Angiogenesis in the morning. Nourishment at night. There the water had a place to run.

Abdul's belly, however, was a vault. A monsoon was in his liver—hepatitis, some malignancy. A few days earlier the hospital an hour away had sent us a report from their lab that his liver enzymes were elevated. We figured that on physical exam. But why? No further tests we could do, no curative treatment to offer. Palliation was obsolete.

When he was thirteen, he started to lose weight. Now seventeen, he was negative space. Bones hung flesh wherein muscle once thrived. Like most of his family—while they lived in Myanmar—he had no access to school or health care, but he could work the fields. Though described by many as nonliterate because he had no official access to school, he could read the Quran with ease. His recitation of its Surahs was exquisite.

On the darkest night of his life, in August 2017, Abdul and his brother fled westward across foreign rice fields. They were backlit by burning villages and the pierced grief of raped mothers and children-in-slaughter. Their family found a home near Hakimpara Camp, Bangladesh.

The morning I met Abdul, his brother had carried him to our clinic hours before it opened. He lay there, cold, on a bamboo bed. Because we had no linens, his friends gave him pieces of clothing to use as sheets. Abdul's abdomen was discordant and quaked a chaotic pace, beats behind his bones. It was a bowl of water furious to settle while prisoner to the corporeal agitation of disease. His genocide had shifted internally, an annihilation of his once-healthy cells.

Abdul spoke limited English and we, no Rohingya. We relied on our interpreter, Nawshad. When asked about pain, Abdul said, "Everywhere." When asked about his family, he smiled. "They are well." When asked about his home, his response was gratitude. He lived with his family in a box of bamboo—poles and thin crosspieces over which an orange tarpaulin hung.

"Now we are safe," said Abdul.

―

Outside Abdul's examination room, I heard the rumble of 120 patients. Many coughed in the morning air. Smoke from tents littered cloudless skies. Cook-fires in the tents suggested that nourishment was available; they also caused chronic cough. Smoke from the fires brought entire families to us suffering respiratory distress. Gentle yet toxic billows from the tents were the new normal.

Abdul told us he lost his appetite three days ago. He said he did not miss dahl and rice, mangos and bananas, though he knew that he should. He had not drunk for a day. I unwrapped an IV cannula and Abdul jumped. It was that quiver we see in our chronically ill patients who, for their entire lives, are stuck with needles. Those patients who we assume won't mind just another shot. But they are the ones who feel the pain the worst as they catastrophize over another stick, their tolerance for that pain significantly diminished. It was as if Abdul, though new to receiving medical care, was a haruspex—a diviner who examines proceedings from animals' digestive processes—who knew that his own gastrointestinal system would invite the onslaught of frequent injections for the rest of his life. He foresaw years of clinically induced pain. He winced when I cleaned his arm with alcohol.

Abdul's fear-cracked groan shook the bed, and his left hand made a fist as I sought a vein. The needle was in a void; there was no flash of blood in the cannula's chamber. *Pause. Let the vessel de-constrict. Let him relax. Let me relax. Nothing.* I moved the needle; Abdul wailed.

Nawshad whispered into my ear, "No blood." Abdul's eyes irrigated the borrowed T-shirt that he used for a pillow. I told him that I would try again. He whimpered but nodded with soft affirmation. Second stick. Nothing. Abdul arched his back off the mat. He looked at me and sniffled. "Vicious."

Saliva stretched from the bottom of his paan-stained teeth to his splintered lower lip. It was mucilaginous from dehydration but aqueous enough to break and bespatter my face when he, a second time, uttered, "Vicious." A third and fourth time with swollen vehemence, "Vicious, vicious!" I set up for another IV. All the while, I imagined places to which we could transfer Abdul that he might receive appropriate care. They would have diagnostics for his hepatomegaly and cachexia. They would have twenty-four-hour staff, teams of nurses and physicians to treat and listen to his life story. The providers would all speak Rohingya. These thoughts were but daydreams. For extraordinary diseases, with extraordinary measures and extraordinary means, there are ways to treat illness. If you are Rohingya, there is nothing.

An interpreter barged into the room. "Three diphtherias here."

We had a makeshift holding unit a few meters away from our

waiting area where we sent any patient with symptoms of diphtheria. Diphtheria had followed the trajectory of forced migration across the Naf River; so too had measles. We waited patiently for cholera. The diphtheria patients could wait. We needed to get this line started first.

Nawshad kept calm and held Abdul's hand while I stretched the tired tourniquet. Abdul yelled, "Vicious!" as the 20-gauge needle ripped open his forearm to find a home in a thirsty vein.

"We're done," I said and secured the line. I put my hand on Abdul's shoulder. "I'm sorry I hurt you."

Nawshad leaned in behind me and said, "He's fine." Abdul whispered, "Vicious."

In the waiting area outside Abdul's room I heard a shuffle of bare feet. In haste, a mother kicked off her slippers and rushed toward registration. She held a three-month-old in her arms. Her arms and the child's arms, face, and head were coated in soot. Her child's eyes were wide. With each breath his head tilted backward. Accessory muscles in the neck teetered his head to pull oxygen into lungs too congested to breath normally. The mother stood with her anxious child but said nothing. She knew the breathing was not right. I grabbed a suction bulb.

*Saline in the nose to loosen the secretions, and then the bulb. Push farther than you think; when the child winces, pull back on your thumb.* The child held his breath at this new sensation. His eyes closed tightly, pressure-sealed tombs; they repelled me. His lip quivered. An open mouth betrayed an imminent cry. No sound, though. Copious, thick sputum was wrenched from his nose. The sound of a ripped paper bag precluded his announcement that he could breathe once again. He howled. His mother exhaled. She then laughed a sigh of relief. We taught her how to use the bulb and what symptoms to watch for in the future to suction him at home. I told her that she could handle this. My interpreter said, "Yes, she can."

Two liters of fluid in, and Abdul looked less pale. His heart rate had decreased from 150 to 120. Slower was better but not good enough. We called to transfer him to a clinic that could rehydrate him overnight.

The afternoon light shifted the sky. Winter's golden-red skies gave us two more hours to work. If we stayed in the camp after sunset the military would arrest us. A translucent brown sheen retched upward from the now dry roads. Overloaded lorries, full of bamboo for new non-permanent homes, choked the thoroughfare. The bamboo would be used up by tomorrow. New tents for a thousand more refugees.

We called for an ambulance—rather, a van with a gurney. It had a rusted oxygen tank tied to the back of the driver's seat with twine. The mask attached to the tank was clouded with memories of dying breaths. Abdul said he could walk the short distance from the clinic to the ambulance. He took five steps on his own and then leaned heavily on his brother and me. The entirety of his bones and youth was in our hands for the last step as we lifted him onto the stained gurney. I put my hand on Abdul's hand. He laid his hand across his abdomen.

One last time he said, "Vicious."

Nawshad closed the door to the ambulance.

"He really liked you," said Nawshad with careless confidence. "All day long he sent you wishes."

---

**TIM CUNNINGHAM** began his health care career as a clown named Dr. Bumble. His work—sharing laughter at Boston Children's Hospital—inspired him to become an emergency nurse. Then a foray in academia and executive leadership landed him a position as a vice president in a large health system in the Southeastern United States. Now a keynote speaker and award-winning author, Cunningham works with teams across the country to keep the art of healing alive in health care.

# 5

# ALONE AGAIN, UNNATURALLY

*Loneliness and Loss*

ESSAY

# Being Seen

## CARA HABERMAN

STARING BLANKLY AT the yellow-and-black checkered gate in front of me, it occurs to me that it is taking a moment too long for the parking attendant to read out my total. I glance up at her and find dark, serious brown eyes searching my face. A jolt of recognition—it's her.

A confession: This is not, in fact, the medical faculty parking deck. My residents call it "Princess Parking," when you pay a few dollars to park in the much closer patient and visitor lot. As a rule-follower by nature, I almost never do this. Only on weekends, when it's nearly empty anyway, and I always wear my jacket zipped up to the neck to hide my scrubs and badge, as if the parking police are going to arrest me.

In fact, the last time I parked here was a few months ago. I remember because it was the end of a particularly exhausting week. I had been up most of the night before speaking with my resident team about an assortment of unusual admissions. My list of patients that morning held the promise of a difficult day, so as I approached the hospital, I gave myself the little treat of a shorter walk by turning into the "Princess Parking" deck.

Indeed, that day spun out as emotionally draining as I anticipated. We told one mother her child most likely had cancer, and we sat and cried with her. We gave another family a life-altering diagnosis for their newborn infant. One of my patients was removed from her mother's custody, and we listened to the accusing wails of a family being torn apart. Knowing it was the safest choice for the child did not make it any easier to hear. Another mother, terrified in the face of her baby's illness and lacking ways to cope, lashed out and verbally abused our team. After a long, tense talk, we managed to regain a fragile trust on both sides.

As is often the case, I did not eat lunch, go to the bathroom, or really even sit down all day. When I walked out of the unit hours later, I was hollowed out, empty. I had given every last bit of myself to the work of the day. When I got to my car I just sat, feeling as gray as the concrete wall in front of me. Eventually my hands remembered how to turn the ignition, my body finding the energy to drive up to the exit gate. I handed the parking attendant my ticket, and for a second, I put my head back against the headrest and closed my eyes. There were tears gathering below the surface, and I quickly blinked them back. I took a deep breath and reached for my wallet.

But as I turned back to the attendant, she was staring intently at me. She cocked her head a little to the side, like a bird, and looked at me another moment. Then without saying a word she raised the gate. I was confused for a moment. With a jut of her chin she signaled, "Go on." Then the tears came, as I was flooded with a tremendous sense of being seen. Here I was holding it together all day long, and this woman saw in the span of a few seconds that I was barely keeping it in and so very much could use a little bit of kindness. "Thank you," I whispered, and I drove on through.

That particular day was months ago. And here we are again, another long day, another searching look from a woman who must watch hundreds of people pass through this gate. I marvel at the deep intensity of her gaze. I imagine her studying each car, calculating how many people she can bestow her benevolence on before it might be noticed. Is she trying to decipher who lost a loved one, who received bad news, who had the worst day? All this goes through my mind in a split second, and I remember that I did not, by those measures, have anywhere close to the worst day. A hard day, to be sure. But not the worst. Someone else may need her gift today. So I summon a little smile, brighten my eyes a bit, say, "Good afternoon."

 Her gaze softens suddenly, then darts away. Her stance shifts from Bountiful Goddess of the Parking Deck to simply Parking Lot B Attendant. "That'll be four dollars please."

---

**CARA HABERMAN** is an associate professor of pediatrics at the Wake Forest School of Medicine in Winston-Salem, North Carolina. She uses narrative medicine to foster compassion and teach others about the heart of medicine.

# Infectious

## DOUG HESTER

The last lightning bug of summer wanders across the Nashville skyline, blinking, seeking a mate to stave off the inevitable, the approach of autumn, the destiny of a lonely demise. The light pulses slowly, flickering within the wind, which caresses the leaves, crackling as they prepare to release.

Somewhere in that skyline, beyond the silhouetted leaves, a physician rounds. She bounces from room to room, examining, listening, explaining, prescribing, healing. My wife wades through the pathogens, who detain her again in the wards tonight.

The metal lattice of her deck chair absorbs the dusk light and grows cool in bright emptiness. The bug wavers above the glowing iron, but continues to blink, flashing into the darkness. Hopeful someone will see him. Hopeful it's not too late in the season.

Hopeful the life he's burning as a message is received.
He hovers near the corner of the house,
and—in a gust—is gone. I soon follow, switching off
the deck light and stepping into a quiet house
as the glow fades.

---

**DOUG HESTER** is an academic anesthesiologist in Nashville, Tennessee, who has an MFA in poetry from Murray State University. His work appears in *JAMA, Anesthesiology, Anesthesia & Analgesia*, and *Chest*.

ESSAY

# Harvest

WILLIAM BACHMAN

WE GOT INTO the car around 11 PM to drive to the eastern part of the state. The senior transplant surgeon drove; the junior surgeon rode shotgun, and they made small talk during the two-hour trip. We two third-year students sat in the back. We were quiet. When we arrived, we went inside and were directed to the operating room. The liver and heart transplant teams from opposite corners of the state were already at work, so we watched and waited.

I had seen kidneys transplanted during our elective, but I'd never experienced their procurement. Several surgeons were hunched over a wide-open abdominal and chest cavity. The rest of the body was not visible; the head was behind the anesthesiologist's drape wall, the legs were covered and inert. The OR scene was typical, but I knew that the goal was not. The space seemed no different from any operating room. It was bright with surgical lights at 1 AM; there was intense activity. There were sponges and bloody gauze on the floor, instrument trays, surgeons cutting and cauterizing, nurses handing and receiving instruments, everyone moving with purpose. New to clinical rotations, I was drawn in by these actions and watched intently, focused on the surgery while anesthetized emotionally. I concentrated on trying to understand the anatomy and the surgical methods used in extracting organs from the body, while I suppressed the true import of what they were doing.

The heart and liver teams finished up and started packing their organs and equipment. They made room for us. Our two surgeons stepped into place, and my friend and I held retractors while they dissected the surrounding tissue and vessels, then painstakingly removed the kidneys, taking care to pack them in ice in the coolers we'd brought.

We students had heard the minimum about this patient's accident when we got the phone call. The donor was a nineteen-year-old who'd had too much to drink with friends and had attempted a back flip off a wall, landing on his head, causing massive brain injury and brain death. That was all. I couldn't process any of that as I studied our surgeons' technique and care, straining to hold the abdominal cavity open and respond to the curt instructions, being a good medical student.

Quiet and obedient. All the thoughts about what exactly we were doing and who we were doing it to felt secondary as we went about the necessary tasks—we were there for organs.

I was a few years older than this kid. I'd done many stupid, drunken things in my life that weren't too far from what he'd done. I'd ended up with a huge swollen ankle and crutches for a couple of weeks after jumping off some stairs, inebriated. I had had other minor injuries, admonishments from police, hangovers. I could've been him. I couldn't think about that.

I wasn't conscious of any of these feelings in the bright operating room filled with surgeons and nurses and techs from different hospitals, extracting life-sustaining parts from this young man to put into others. Taking this rare opportunity to benefit the living.

Our surgeons finished up. The chief told me to close the patient's long neck-to-pubis incision, emphasizing that I was to do a good job. He watched me for a bit, had me take out and redo several stitches until he was sure I wasn't going to screw up, then left me to finish. Though I was tired, I took care. I felt a responsibility to make sure his incision was clean and aligned for his funeral.

As I was finishing up, the activity of cleaning the operating rooms had already started. Staff were straightening up, picking up debris, removing dressings and drapes from the body, taking instrument trays away, closing drawers, preparing to sweep and sterilize the floors and surface for the next case. We gathered our gear and coolers, the surgeons said goodbye to their colleagues, and it was time for us to drive back. Our attending doctors told me and my fellow student to meet them at the car, then turned and went outside.

I started to leave but I stopped. I turned around and looked back from the doorway at the operating room for a long moment. The young man was now entirely visible; his face, arms and legs, torso, all of him, uncovered. He was spread out on the table, blotched with dried betadine and blood, lifeless, incised, alone. And in that brief span when I stood there, I was able to see. I saw a young man at the start of his life, having friends and family, maybe a partner, possibly hopes and dreams and likely no thoughts of mortality. I was able to feel. I felt what I couldn't while we took his organs and finalized the end of his life. I felt an overwhelming sadness, a deep grief over the loss of this person, his connections, his needs and ambitions, his loves. I felt shame over my actions, the failure to acknowledge his sacrifice with the proper reverence it deserved while we harvested. I can't have remained at the door for more than a few seconds. Yet I still see that young man and feel that hole where his life should have been, thirty years later.

Now, like a smell that can transport one instantly back in time to another place, some hospitalized patients I care for who are beyond help and who are anonymous to me trigger something that immediately brings me back to that doorway, and that scene, and that sorrow and regret.

All I could do in that long moment was helplessly bear witness, something I'd failed to do while we swarmed over him and extracted what was needed. In an operating room one hundred miles from my medical school, after an organ harvest in the middle of the night from a brain-dead young man, I stood there and looked, and saw, and felt.

There was absolutely nothing I could do except that. I paused, and then I left.

We drove in silence and arrived back at 4 AM. We students were entrusted to deliver the two coolers with the kidneys to the surgery suite, and then we had a couple of hours to sleep while the transplant recipient arrived and was prepped for his surgery.

I've never seen a harvest since.

---

**WILLIAM BACHMAN** is a cardiologist at a medical college in upstate New York. He has been in clinical practice for twenty-seven years and has learned much from being an educator. His teaching experiences have emphasized the importance of listening and treating patients, and each other, with kindness and respect.

SHORT STORY

# Late

I. CORI BAILL

LATE AT NIGHT, a long time ago, when Sandi was an OB/GYN intern, before electronic health records and much use of personal electronic devices, back when a beeper was a big deal and when it was rare for anyone in Baltimore to have one unless a doctor or a drug dealer, Sandi was a night owl. Others in her residency class happily woke early every morning. Then, at the first long shadow of the day, they were ready to find any soft corner, or even a not-so-soft spot, for a nap. Not Sandi. That was when she felt the lethargy of the day lift—as if sunshine and daylight were thick blankets to be tossed aside. She felt enlivened as the day retreated. Her step lightened and her posture eased.

In those days every hospital ward had chart carts. They resembled the book carts that to this day inhabit library stacks. The four-wheeled gray metal chart carts had large rubber wheels and were put to hard work like so many mine mules. In the fluorescent glow of the late shift, when the generously proportioned night nurses began unwrapping their various bags and boxes of supper and treats and poured drinks brought from home from their thermoses, when rustles and crinkles accompanied their shared dinner and gossip, Sandi filled an empty gray cart with her patients' five-ring blue vinyl–bound charts. Back then there was no dictation service for the residents, no Dictaphones, no tablets. They used pen and paper. She selected the cart least used and least likely to be missed due to a wonky left wheel. She was pleased it no longer squeaked, thanks to a stray can of WD-40 she had found in the back of a janitorial closet. While the other residents scribbled away in the last of the day, Sandi never had.

Instead, later, when night had settled, and shadows had disappeared into the darkness, she and her cart would career down the hall of the gyn-oncology ward. There, finding a family sitting vigil, she wished them a good evening. She'd point to the charts and say, "I have hours of work here. Go home and shower. Change your clothes. I'll stay with your Aunt Noreen" (or a sister named Millie, or a mother named June . . .). And she did.

Many times, a whisper slipped from one or two of the group as they stirred and gathered sweaters or fleeces, purses and magazines. "How much longer?" they would ask.

"She's suffering," they would say. "Help her," they might plead.

Sandi always promised to do what she could to keep their loved one comfortable. "But that is all I can do." She said this clearly and firmly while wrestling her cart into the room. She settled herself in the hard plastic hospital-issue recliner next to the bed and, pulling a chart from the rack, began to write.

She knew a simple truth, one that spoke to her as did the night. Her presence was a comfort that came with no ties. Patients, she had observed, even those deeply unresponsive, those with only a toe remaining in the mortal world, avoided departing in the bustle of the day, doubly so when a loving vigil crowded the room and engulfed their soul like a snug camisole.

She imagined that it weighed just enough to tether that last small digit of their being. So, Sandi came late in the night to keep uncomplicated company while scribbling through one chart after another, occasionally flipping from section to section to check a lab or to look up a study.

She sat quietly by the beloved's bed. Sometimes she sat by the bed of one alone but unlikely to recover yet hanging on night after night. They, she thought, might be afraid to take the final step from this world all alone. She was unsurprised when, as she paged through charts, a patient would slip away.

Hours later, rarely more than two or three, the family returned. Most often they were filled with gratitude that the final vigil had ended. "Thank you," they would say as she wheeled the wonky cart out the door. One or another might add, "We won't say what you did." Often a hug or a clasped hand was offered. It might even be a night nurse who thanked her, rounding after supper was packed away. She never bothered to explain that there was nothing to tell.

---

**I. CORI BAILL** is a professor of obstetrics and gynecology at the University of Central Florida College of Medicine, in Orlando. Her areas of interest include menopausal medicine and medical education, and she is a career-long supporter of Planned Parenthood. She received a Certification of Professional Achievement in narrative medicine from Columbia University. In addition to her short stories, Baill is the author of the picture book *Why is Mommy Crying? Explaining early pregnancy loss to young children.*

POEM

# The Doctor's White Room

SUMIT PARIKH

Every day
this room
devours
the sun
the sweet
sweet air

And still
licks its
empty
lips
tasting
more
despair

Every
morning
I walk in

with
someone
new
and close
the door



**SUMIT PARIKH** is a poet from Cleveland whose work is shaped by his experiences as a pediatric neurologist, son, and father. He finds poetry in both the delicate complexities of his work as a physician and the quiet moments of everyday family life. His work has appeared in *I-70 Review, North Dakota Quarterly*, and *The Marbled Sigh*. Read more of his work at sumitspoetry.com.

ESSAY

# Invisible

JOANNE WILKINSON

I AM APPROACHING the bedside of a sixty-two-year-old woman with Alzheimer's dementia, whose disease has become so advanced that in recent weeks she cannot speak or make any of her needs known. She had been conveyed finally to a nursing home so her family, exhausted from months of heroic care, could get a break. At the nursing home she promptly developed bedsores and sepsis, went from there to the ICU, and has now come out to my team on the med-surg floor, where we are planning a family meeting to discuss hospice.

The woman in the bed is ten years older than I am. When I was in grade school, she was in high school. When I was in high school, she was newly finished with college. I had cassette tapes and she had eight-tracks. She probably listened to Carole King, and Bread. She's not that much older than I am and certainly doesn't seem old enough to be here, in this bed, for no reason other than bad luck, about to be transferred to hospice to die.

She is very small, frail even, with a deeply lined face and a scraggle of gray hair. Would I look this way with no hair salon and no makeup? Instead of a "sitter," as we call the nursing assistants that do overtime shifts alongside the patients who present a safety risk, she has an AvaSys, which is the remote electronic version of the sitter, a benign robot elegantly posed in the corner overlooking her bed. Somewhere, on some screen, people can watch me interact with her as I steal up to the side of her bed.

She is wearing huge mitts, like boxing gloves, the adult version of those little mittens babies wear so they won't scratch their eyes with their fingernails. Her hospital bed is a tangle of sterile-looking white sheets and one of those white hospital waffle-knit blankets. Down by her feet, there is an unexpected addition: a large stuffed bunny, white, with long loping ears trailing over the edge of the bed, tipped over slightly and leaning toward the window.

I don't think she can really hear me, or really appreciate who I am and what this is about. I don't make a big effort to explain things to her or tell her I'm the doctor in charge. Better that I remain mostly invisible. "Hi," I say softly. "I'm one of the doctors, just here to listen to your heart." I pull out my stethoscope. "Look at your sweet bunny," I add. "I'm going to move him up here so you can be a little bit closer, okay? I think he's lonely." I tuck the bunny next to her forearm, so that the part of her skin that's uncovered can feel his soft furry belly. "You rest, okay?" This is what I always say to patients who are very ill or dying—you rest, to the intubated ICU patient who I don't think can hear me; you rest, to the confused and agitated elderly patient who is at the end of their life. I hope that in some small corner of their brain, it reminds them of a time when they were ill as a child and their mom tucked them in on the couch with a tray and some grape Tylenol and a TV dinner. You rest, she might have said to them as she laid a cool hand on their forehead, and then I hope they slid into a nap knowing that when they woke, they would be feeling better.

I sneak away from the bed after only being with her for maybe ninety seconds, but there is nothing really for me to do here. Nothing I appreciate or notice about her physical exam is going to change the fact that she can't swallow, is malnourished and only intermittently conscious. As I am approaching the Purell station to sanitize my hands, I look back for a moment and see, to my surprise, that she has turned her head, slowly, to regard the bunny, now sitting straight up next to her shoulder so he can make eye contact.

In the hallway, two more patients to see, my step falters for a moment as I wonder where all the acts of kindness go—the soup, the nurses helping people lie down more comfortably, the extra blankets, the straw to drink water when lying down. Sure, some patients get better and clasp our hands as they are wheeling out, fully dressed in street clothes, to the door. Some send a cookie tray after they recover. But some, like this patient, merely die, and we are left not knowing whether any of it made a difference, really, which kind of makes me wonder what I have been doing with my whole life. I thought, when I became a doctor, that one day I would know the answers, but more and more I feel I am just making motions on the sidelines of other people's tragedies, and maybe not affecting them in any meaningful way.

I rub my Purell'd hands together more and more rapidly, willing myself not to look back at the bunny, and my stride starts to speed up so I can finish rounds on time.

---

**JOANNE WILKINSON** is an associate professor of family medicine at Brown University, a voracious reader, and a single parent who writes whenever she gets the chance.

ESSAY

# Calluses

## LAURA B. VATER

I'M SIXTEEN, AND my hands are covered in thick, hardened layers of skin across my upper palms—my body's attempt at protecting me from the repetitive friction of the uneven bars. When they're particularly dry, I soak them in warm water, cover them with a copious amount of emollient, and sleep in plastic gloves.

At practice, I press white chalk into my hands before fastening the leather grips around my wrists and over my middle and ring fingers. Then I spray the fabric with water, use a wire brush to gently roughen the surface, and apply another generous layer of chalk. Despite all these protective measures, a sharp, stinging pain soars through my left hand as I circle the high bar. It's a dreaded *rip*—the round callus has torn open, and the blood trickles over my palm and onto my plum purple leotard.

After washing and bandaging the wounded skin, I transition to the balance beam, trying my best to keep going. The sore takes weeks to heal.

Nowadays, my hands are mostly callus-free, but my career comes with a different sort of repetitive strain. As a medical oncologist caring for patients with advanced gastrointestinal cancers, nearly eighty percent of my patients die from their illnesses, and the work is emotionally taxing. No, that's not even a close approximation. The work is often gut-wrenchingly heartbreaking.

Caring for about sixty patients a week, it's a routine part of my job to tell someone they have incurable cancer and support them during the distress that follows. Then I guide them through the difficult events that often ensue: side effects from treatment, progression of disease, anticipatory grief, increasing dependence on others, and—eventually—death. Sometimes, an extra layer of devastation blankets an already painful situation—a spouse divorces a patient after diagnosis, or a single parent faces the prospect of leaving behind a young child.

In training, I often felt crushed by the weight and wondered how this career could be sustainable. By observing my physician teachers, I learned techniques to blunt my emotions until I could step into a bathroom, call room, or stairwell to cry. Once, while witnessing a college student with end-stage cancer calmly grapple with the decision about hospice, I'd had to read the caution sign on an exam chair over and over to keep myself from sobbing.

I quickly learned that how I processed and coped with this lingering grief was just as important as mastering the clinical skills of medicine. Like the grips and chalk of my youth, I reached for tools to help buffer the stress and mitigate compassion fatigue: journaling, therapy, meditation, exercise, and books that offered temporary respite. On especially tough days, I'd remind myself that I didn't cause my patients' illnesses, nor could I control the outcomes of their treatments.

Several years into my career now, my emotional reactivity has lessened, but my muted internal responses sometimes fill me with guilt.

Recently, I told a patient that his newly diagnosed gastric cancer was more advanced than we had previously thought. The scans showed metastases in the liver, and surgery was no longer an option. The patient's wife shrieked out in grief, and the resident next to me was visibly distraught, wiping away tears. I also felt sad and wished they weren't facing this, but the pain did not wreck me. I wondered if the resident thought I was uncaring, and a flash of shame passed through me.

I left the room, let out a sigh, and went to see the next patient, because that is what this work requires.

On the drive home, the shame resurfaced. Had I become hardened? I knew that an emotional callus had formed from the strain of the work, but was *I* callous?

The words were so similar. An online search revealed that both come from the Latin *callosus*, meaning hard-skinned or tough. It's where the thick bundle of nerve fibers separating the brain's hemispheres—the corpus callosum—gets its name. I scrolled through the examples and stared at one in horror: *The doctor seemed callous when delivering the news.* Was this how I appeared to my patient and his wife?

I flashed back to a statistic my mentor once told me: I'd share bad news with patients ten to thirty thousand times in my career. Living this reality now, I realize it's simply not possible to take on every patient's pain. I'm one person, and my energy and capacity are not infinite. There will be times I must lean back to preserve my well-being, function in my role, and compassionately support my patients through the challenges of illness.

As hard as it is to accept that my emotional responses have changed, part of me is grateful for this layer of mental armor. Just as calluses enable gymnasts to perform incredible feats on the bars, emotional calluses allow us to remain present for life's most anguishing events when others might turn away. Understanding this has helped me release some of the shame.

The truth is, rips still happen. Often unexpectedly.

I'm thirty-six and standing at my desk in clinic. My next patient is just a few years older than me and has four small children. She's been through intensive chemotherapy and surgery for her pancreatic cancer, and her scan report pops up. Holding my breath, I double-click: she has new tumors in her lungs and liver indicative of metastatic, incurable disease.

As I walk to her room, my muscles tense. She and her husband look at me expectantly, then crumple as I speak the unspeakable.

"But my kids," she sobs. "They're just babies."

A pang wallops my chest as I sit with her, and a tear rolls down my face. When she asks for a hug, I wrap her in one.

At home, my mind turns to her while eating dinner with my family, and then again while trying to fall asleep. How much more time will the treatments give her? I think of her children growing up without their mom. Will the littlest be too young to remember her?

In reality, no matter how much our bodies may try to insulate us from the pain, it's impossible to do this work without being affected. Rips are part of the deal. Perhaps the only hint of relief in all this comes from knowing I still have soft spots.

The next week, she comes to the clinic for treatment, and I softly knock on the door.

After we discuss the risks and benefits, she tells me it's her daughter's fourth birthday.

"I hope I'm here to celebrate the next one." Her voice cracks, and her husband slides his hand into hers.

"Me too," I say, my eyes filling with water. "I'll be with you every step of the way."

In the hallway, I take an extra moment to collect myself before looking at my list. There are rooms filled with other patients who need my care, presence, and attention, some of whom I'm meeting for the first time. With a long exhale, I try to release some of the ache, then walk to the next patient's room.

I'll do my best to keep going.

---

**LAURA B. VATER** is a medical oncologist in Indianapolis, a writer, and a TEDx and commencement speaker. Her narrative writing has been featured in several medical journals, and she is working on her first novel. Read more at lauravater.com.

ESSAY

# The Idea of Him

H. READE JOO

An antidote to the despair of romantic loss is to tell yourself or your friends: It wasn't him, it was the time and the place; it was the night, the summertime, the mountains, the gondola. It was the cool lake water you loved, and the leaves just changing. It wasn't him, but your mood that week, the layered coincidences of train schedules and assigned seats conspiring. In other words, desire is of your own making. Nothing was truly lost. It wasn't him; it was the idea of him.

For example, a friend goes on a single dinner date and imagines a happy future together based on little evidence, ignoring many details of her dining partner, then is devastated when there is no second date. The sadness at a relationship's end may be more about the loss of companionship, not the specific person or a unique chemistry you shared. I have always thought serious attention is required to feel love that is specific, love that is true. I would assure myself that only a particular kind of person moved me, even when it was not true, and make lists of would-be meaningful attributes and experiences. This view defended against the pain of loss—including the agony of finding myself in the depth of a relationship without affection.

At their prenatal appointments, mothers and fathers talk about how excited they are to meet their newborns. I have been in the room when many of these first joyful meetings happened, sometimes after long and difficult labors. One night I was in obstetric triage. A woman came in because she hadn't felt her baby kicking as much as the previous day. From outside the room, I heard her say that her due date was the next morning. She felt silly coming in now, but she and her husband just wanted to check. He sat beside their hospital delivery bag.

She smiled at him over her huge belly while she had an ultrasound.

The nurse didn't leave the room for a long time. Then she called for our attending. "I couldn't find a heartbeat," she said. "Would you like to try?" We all knew what it meant: She hadn't had any difficulty finding the heart. Our attending went in. At my workstation, just outside the room, I heard what I thought was a woman laughing. As it grew louder, I expected I would soon hear a second voice, of another person telling jokes to make her laugh. I didn't. I soon recognized it was not laughter at all but wailing as I'd never heard before in public. I heard her sob for an hour. At the nurses' station we all cried as we worked—for a patient we hadn't met, who had lost a baby she had never met. Later that night, she delivered. The cord had been wrapped three times around the baby's neck.

Parents say, "We are so excited to meet you," but if this meeting is like any other, it's like meeting a neighbor in the apartment next door, whose schedule and favorite songs and coffee order you've already learned over the months of living so near. But the meeting is not like any other. The baby had hands, and he curled in one direction, not the other.

Sometimes, a love can pre-date its object. The idea of a person, pre-formed, settles around its match. An affection developed over years in the imagination is felt, in a train car or hospital room, to be instantaneous. When a friend asks me, "How soon can I know if this love is real?" I respond, "I think it is real." This form of love can be sustained for years. Object and context are inseparable. A great love can exist largely in the imagination. Perhaps this is the reason new parents sometimes say, in front of each other and in total agreement, that they never felt love so pure and powerful as when they first held their child.

Instead of saying, "You only love the idea of him," know that is the proof you are capable of feeling love, proof that you will feel it again. I say it not in defense, but in hope. Your grief will subside. The idea of him is the hardest loss to bear.

---

**H. READE JOO** studied neuroscience at Johns Hopkins University as an undergraduate, completed a research year as a Churchill Scholar at the University of Cambridge, then finished medical and neuroscience training at the School of Medicine, University of California, San Francisco. Joo is now a research-track psychiatry resident at Stanford University studying the anthropology of maternity and psychiatry, and the neurophysiology of memory.

# 6

# THE PLAGUE YEARS

*Fear and Panic*

ESSAY

# The Shape of the Shore

RANA AWDISH

In April our bodies stopped pretending.

Standing at the glass door of the ICU room, fear set the rate and depth of our breath—rapid and shallow. We were desperate to capture the small, trapped pockets of clean air behind our masks. Our hearts ached from hurling themselves against our sternums. Our pulses bounded in our throats with a dry and weary urgency.

Our bodies were warning us; we were not okay.

Our coworkers walked us to get tested for the virus. They would also gently encourage us to decorate our PPE. We'd find brightly colored markers and puffy paint set out for us. As if by brightening the black face shields we could lighten the cloud of anxious dread we carried into every room.

The psychologists made more formal, ceremonial suggestions. We could create a kind of meaningful ritual around the donning of our protective equipment, they explained.

*You could attempt to acknowledge the sacredness of the act of applying protection to your bodies. Take a moment to try to envision an invisible cloak of bright white light enveloping you in safety. Picture carrying that safe, comforting blanket of protection with you into the rooms.*

We stared back blankly, seeing only the desperate thrashing patients on the other side of the glass. We wondered if we were the only ones who could see them.

At a time when no one could ensure our safety, we could color and pretend. Or we could choose to care for our patients.

We would learn to live with airlessness; we would learn to do the work while holding our breath.

---

When two twenty-year-old patients died in rapid succession, we had to leave the unit. We needed distance from the sticky blood on the floor. We needed not to see the passive drape of their arms off the sides of the gurneys, their painted nails and supplicant posturing still silently begging us to save them. We walked away, shaking and nauseated. It wasn't a choice. Our bodies knew to rescue us from the scene.

But the administration felt we had saved ourselves the wrong way. Needing our eyes to see something alive or even the sky, needing to hear something other than agonal breaths signaled a problem. Our action had revealed some dispositional property about us; that like glass we were predisposed to breaking. In attempting to protect ourselves, we had validated the concerns about our frailty.

They brought in experts to explain us to ourselves.

*A panic attack is a sudden episode of fear that triggers an intense physical reaction, even when there is no real danger.*

But there was real danger. We were appropriately terrified. We took issue with their terminology. When the psychologists framed our experiences in terms of depression and anxiety and PTSD, we withdrew, feeling unheard and misread. What we were experiencing was not a diagnosis, it was a tragedy.

Our capacity may have been overwhelmed, like small boats caught in a sudden sea swell. But we knew our little boats were solid. Our vessels should not be blamed; they would withstand it.

---

The psychologists wore professional clothes and readjusted their new, blue surgical masks frequently. They positioned themselves in the outermost ring of chairs and had to lean toward us when they spoke. They wondered if they should be wearing scrubs. We thought it unnecessary, in a conference room, removed from patients. We didn't recognize ourselves as patients.

Staring at the endless twisted waves of blue industrial carpet on the ground, we listened mostly to each other, which felt just like listening to versions of ourselves from other units on other floors.

"I don't recognize myself anymore. I don't know who I am here," a nurse began, her face emotionless.

"I kept a mother from her baby. I didn't allow her to nurse. I had to treat her as if she was a threat to her own child. And when the mother cried, I thought she was being so short-sighted. It was only for a few days until she tested negative. I remember thinking she was so selfish." We shook our heads at our own admission.

*It's useful conceptually to think of spheres of control. While we can't change our circumstances, we can change our response to them. That's the sphere where we have room for choice and personal agency.*

"A choice. What kind of a person is so afraid of their own patient they don't immediately run in to help them? I watched my patient suffocate through the window," we accused ourselves, while admitting it was true.

In the minutes it took to put our PPE on, we had watched our patients die. In a quiet side reaction, we felt the good things leave our body, and grief come to stay.

We leaned forward and bowed our heads in order to redirect the flow of tears. We couldn't risk touching our faces and we need them to fall onto our scrubs. We couldn't ruin our masks.

---

The absence of family made the care feel somehow invisible and hollow. Families didn't attend the births. They couldn't stand with us at the bedside of the dying. If they came in, they faced mandatory quarantine, and they would lose their already tenuous jobs.

They could spread disease to vulnerable members of the family. There was no actual choice.

Excluded, families couldn't know what we knew. We knew their father had already crossed a threshold. The machines and drugs were maintaining a kind of physiologic existence, but the father they knew would never return.

In this place, our language failed us. "He's about the same today. No real change," didn't mean what we wished it meant. We didn't know how to explain that stability was really inertia and there was no force we could apply to that body that would shock it out of rest.

Though we applied energy and chemicals to try to change them from dead to less dead or not dead, we couldn't reach their threshold.

The shocks reverberated through their bodies and were absorbed by ours.

"I was in the room alone, shocking him six or seven times while I waited for the team to gown up. He was so dead and I was shocking him again and again, and it felt like torture," we said.

"It feels very harmful. I felt inhuman," we said.

We were admitting what was true. We had crossed nearly every line that had defined us. We had done harm. With more waves headed in, more harm would certainly follow. We would have to endure whatever came.

---

On the outside, we had trouble relating to our own families.

Our children needed help with multiplication tables and planning virtual field trips. The absurdity of planning a hypothetical three-day road trip, across a plague-infested state, when travel was banned, felt intentionally cruel. No one seemed to understand how little remained of us. Our spouses worried about supplies of paper towels and complained of Zoom fatigue.

In our absence, the news and our neighbors had labeled it a war. We read it as an attempt to keep us cordoned in the infected city while they remained sheltered in their suburban nests. A wall intended to strengthen the perimeter. And because war is mostly myth, all they had to do was hold up ideals that seemed worthy of the level of human sacrifice that they knew would be required of us. They hung white ribbons on our own trees and doors, as if we had already gone missing.

They invoked their God. "We've seen you, heroes. You're doing God's work. You are His hands."

At times, we invoked our God. In the other place we believed more, or we needed to believe more. "God didn't put me here, at this bedside, just to allow me to be harmed. My PPE is my protection yes, but He is my protection," we said.

We knew we could still die.

There were unexpected surrogates for our grief on the outside. When the evening news reported that a woman was killed in a shark attack off the coast of Maine, we turned from the TV in tears, aching for the family who watched helplessly as she died in the water. Hearing that they had stood by on the shoreline and did not go into the water validated us somehow. They knew what would happen if they went in. Their helplessness wrecked us.

Our days intruded into our dreams. We were at the beach by the steep cliffs. The dark sand was covered in half-drowned people, and we had to pull them to safety before the next wave crashed or they'd be swept away. When the tide receded, it left piles of rocks that we'd stack and restack endlessly, to track the number of bodies we'd lost.

At night we knew our small boats had already struck the rocks and we were taking on water. We would be pulled underneath the surface. The only question was when.

―

In the room with the psychologists, we spent our time turning things over, examining the facets of our dark, internal kaleidoscopes. We held up reflections of our pain and found they were just distorted projections about the healers we thought we should be.

*I want you to remember other difficult times in your past and how impossible it seemed to survive them. Bad times, like a relationship ending, and how it felt like the end of the world at the time. Just like with that, you'll come through this stronger.*

We tried to imagine being the sort of people who felt like a breakup was the end of the world. Instead of sadness, we were only able to conjure a lightness of being. There were dresses there and mascara that ran when we cried. Long dinners and chilled cocktails that made us giggle. We had none of those things here.

Sometimes, the psychologists' affirmations made our own words stick in our chests. The shame felt too real to verbalize. So we wrote the terrible things down on yellow sticky notes. We passed them to the outside of the circle and the psychologists imbricated them, layer by layer, on poster board as if they were helping us to build something from the paper tiles.

We turned in a paper that said, "People don't understand, there are things worse than death. I feel guilty for hoping the patients will choose death."

When the psychologists read the notes back to us, sighing, we replied to ourselves, "You know, it's okay to hope for peace, in any form that it may take."

"His daughter couldn't bring herself to come in alone, so she asked me to take a picture of her dad's body for her. I didn't know if it was okay. I opened the blinds, and I straightened the sheets, and I said a prayer, and I took it. I'd never done that before," we said. We texted pictures of the dead from this place.

We offered ourselves an alternative reflection: "You gave her what she needed to grieve. There is meaning in that."

"We used to leave the room when the family would say their goodbyes. It felt sacred, and private. Now I stand there stupidly, holding the iPad, and I don't want to have to be the only human contact they have at the end of their life. I am the last humanity they have access to, and I don't want to be with them. It's too much," we said.

"It is too much," we acknowledged. "But do you hear who you rose to become? In an impossible circumstance, you filled a need that would have been a void."

"That's the thing, I don't know that I actually did anything," we said. "You did so much," we said.

And as we said it, we believed it was solidly true of them.

—

In the silence between our disclosures, we knew we were all the same. Whatever was said next could be said by any one of us.

"There were two men, and I can't get them out of my head. They both asked to call their wives because they knew they were going to die. And I told them, 'No, you can't think like that. We're going to help you.' And those men, they spent those last minutes taking care of their families. They told their wives when bills came in, what the passwords were."

We knew what those men said next. We could still hear echoes of their warbled, drowning voices saying, "I'm not coming out from under this, you won't hear my voice again."

Their final words were anchored in our bodies, and we knew that the iron weight of our collective memory could easily pull us under.

Those two men died in the exact same bed. We couldn't help them.

*You helped them to leave this earth feeling like they had done what they could to care for their families.*

We shook our heads, knowing it was a lie.

One of the men had a disabled, dependent daughter. We knew he died in despair, wondering what would become of his family.

*You helped him do what he could. That's all any of us can do.*

"It's just a helpless feeling," we said. "I don't know what to do with that . . . with that feeling."

"It's the thing we share, and that no one understands, really," we said.

*You could try to leave some of it here.*
We nodded, knowing that we had no other choice.

Alone, it was impossible to reconcile our sense of self with our actions. But together, we learned to set down all the lines we had crossed. We learned we could arrange them end to end and deliberately form a circle out of them. A circle we could step inside and gather within. Of all the tools we were offered there, it was time and space and each other that allowed us to reconstitute ourselves.

In the circle, we saw that the actions we had characterized as inhuman were understandable, even necessary, when set down between us. We saw the sincere intentions of our colleagues. We saw that they were full of goodness, and thought it was possible that we were too.

It seemed to us, sometimes, that we were standing on some shore, watching a version of ourselves being lost to a faceless danger hidden in the waves. But other times, we'd gathered the strength to be able, together, to pull the body to the shore.

In the hallways now, when we raise our arms to wave, we're reminded of those awkward strokes trying to reach each other in the water. Slipping our bodies underneath heavy torsos to raise each other up. Reaching our arms across each other's chests and gripping under armpits to join together. Quieting flailing limbs with our presence. Using our imperfect strengths to bring each other above the surface.

We know now, from this side of it, that it was our breath that allowed us to save each other.

---

**RANA AWDISH** is a pulmonary and critical care physician working in Detroit. Her narrative nonfiction writing includes *In Shock*, a critically acclaimed, bestselling memoir based on her own critical illness. Her newest book is *After Shock*. She is also a visual artist who believes in the healing power of art, often using oil painting to process her experiences.

## My First Mask Was a White Coat

LAUREN FIELDS

I get lost
between my screen
the notes on my paper
the people waiting in rooms,
and my team—
where I barely see
my own brown reflection.

On rounds, names become
numeric, identifiers
saying nothing
of life or story, dim beacons
of a vanishing objective,
and this feels like the last moment
I will notice the shift.

Somewhere in my mind
a code is still
a word you use to enter
treehouses, to commune
in a meaningful meaninglessness
with people you desperately want
to trust.

*Am I becoming
something unfamiliar?*
I want to ask. Instead

I exchange pleasantries
with the man in 421 as if
no one had ever died
in that room before,
as if no one ever would.

---

**LAUREN FIELDS** is a psychiatrist-in-training, and poetry has been an important part of her medical education. Her poems have appeared in the *Healing Muse*, *A Garden of Black Joy: Global Poetry from the Edges of Liberation and Living*, and *Corona: An Anthology of Poems*. In 2020 she tied for second place in the international Hippocrates Health Professionals Award for Poetry, supported by Britain's Fellowship of Postgraduate Medicine.

ESSAY

# Everything

SIMONE BLASER

Tears well and I breathe quickly into my N95 mask. Shouts echo down the hallway. Mr. G has coded during morning rounds. It is the first week of April 2020. Thousands of patients in intensive care units across different hospitals in different cities and different countries have a single diagnosis. With this single diagnosis, a tsunami of patients, hospitals underprepared, staff overworked. With it, a tsunami of death, and desperate families who beg us to do everything to save their loved ones.

Everything—that's the word they always use.

I have been working in the intensive care unit, and many times this past week I have returned to the literature I studied before becoming a physician. There's the line from Thomas Mann's novella *Death in Venice*, when, at the onset of a cholera epidemic, the main character has "a feeling . . . that the world was undergoing a dreamlike alienation, becoming increasingly deranged and bizarre." Only the unreality of fiction can describe the reality of this week, and the line has been in and out of my head like a refrain.

Our own world has undergone a dreamlike alienation, increasingly bizarre and deranged. In medical school we study the role of touch in establishing diagnosis, in building physician–patient trust and mother–child bond—but this highly infectious virus precludes all human contact. Only one physician performs a physical examination each day. We group medicine administrations with blood draws to decrease nursing exposure. The patients are tucked away out of reach, isolated from the hospital ward and the world beyond.

The families beg us to do everything, but our ignorance vastly outweighs our knowledge. There haven't been sufficient randomized controlled trials, the gold standard for medical decision making. The disease is too new. We are bushwhacking, basing treatment decisions on hearsay or on anecdotal reports or on theories of how the body breaks down in response to disease. Low-dose intravenous blood thinners, steroids, hydroxychloroquine—so much the focus of the press—none of it seems to help, but still we administer it. We, too, are desperate. We turn patients facedown to let gravity pull open diseased lung tissue, so clogged with dead cells and fluid that no space remains for oxygen to enter and carbon dioxide to exit. This maneuver seems to help, except when it doesn't. Some patients indeed need less supplemental oxygen while they lie prone. But other patients, with bodies so ravaged by disease, deteriorate further with the flip on their bellies. Sometimes they die.

We practice medicine with humility, urgency, and fear.

Rounds in the ICU now feel as if they've been crafted by Samuel Beckett. The patients are all middle-aged men who presented to the hospital with respiratory symptoms, developed respiratory failure, and now lie in the ICU paralyzed and sedated to tolerate the machines that breathe for them. Eventually their kidneys will fail, and they will require medication to maintain their blood pressure. Every morning we walk up and down the narrow hallway of the ICU, weaving our rolling computers in and around the ventilators and IV poles, stepping over wires and stopping outside each patient's room. Just outside the door, we discuss the patient tucked away within. His story, his recent blood work, his imaging and medications. We make a plan. The plan is the same for all the patients, every day, and essentially what it all amounts to is: watch and wait. On occasion, beeps and alarms and shouts emerge over the basal mechanical hum of the ICU, the only punctuation to the macabre sameness. This new cacophony signals a patient's rapid deterioration. Three patients have died in the last four days.

---

*Asystole, asystole!* The familiar shouts interrupt us as we conduct rounds this morning. Mr. G's heart has stopped and my own heart races as we scramble to his room to evaluate him. His family, like all of the families, has asked for everything.

Before April, when we knew the diseases, our conversations about code status centered on patients' values given our understanding of their prognoses. What makes a patient's life meaningful? How does she imagine her death? Are his values compatible with chest compressions or with a breathing tube? Are his values compatible with lifelong dialysis should his kidneys fail? If her body needs longer than two weeks to heal from the ravages of her disease, are her values compatible with a throat incision through which we would insert a breathing tube?

But now our poor understanding of who survives this new disease hinders our ability to guide these decisions. On most days, I wonder if less is more. Few interventions seem to work by the time patients land in the ICU, and each intervention feels like an added torment for the comatose, with no way for them to accept or decline invasive measures. "Nothing happens, nobody comes, nobody goes, it's awful!" Estragon says to Pozzo in *Waiting for Godot*. Nothing to be done. Perhaps the disease has already passed the point of no return. I haven't seen a single patient survive, though I've heard that elsewhere they do.

Now we conduct these crucial conversations about care by telephone with family members who are not permitted to sit vigil at bedside and witness the deterioration of their loved ones but only to receive news of it. They do not see their loved ones swollen with fluid from kidneys that no longer urinate; they do not see blue hands or facial bruises from spending sixteen hours a day prone.

We reach Mr. G's room and stop outside. The monitor has a flat line. Overnight his blood pressure had plummeted. Four different blood pressure medications snake into the room from the hallway beyond. The medication pumps have been moved to the hallway, to allow the nurses to adjust the drip rates without an additional exposure to Mr. G.

When families ask for everything, I think about religion, how belief in miracles is central to the faith of many. I wonder if asking for less than everything—asking for anything less than full code—is an acknowledgment no miracle will occur. Is that ask tantamount to loss of faith? When the families ask for everything, I understand this choice and I respect it. But sometimes I wonder if those wishes might change were they permitted to visit the hospital, to witness the surreal comatose body, now bloated and bruised, perhaps only tenuously linked to the vibrant loved one they picture. Would they beg us to stop, to let their loved ones die in peace? Would they pray harder?

*He's gone*, my attending says. I peer at him through the glass doors. He looks no different than he did when I visited him yesterday: his swollen body, enveloped in sallow skin, alone with his buzzing and beeping machines. I stare at my feet. There's nothing more we can do. He's maxed on pressors. His kidneys have failed. Chest compressions won't bring him back. He's gone. We nod. The mask pinches my cheeks. He's gone. I'm breathing fast and my chest heaves. Someone told me once that trying to understand death was like looking directly at the sun—indeed, it is blinding. Time of death: 9:34 AM.

We observe a moment of silence. I slip away to the bathroom to cry. I anticipate the relief when, just after I wash my hands, I will remove the mask. I soap up and start to count to twenty. I lose count and start again from one. I wonder if my runny nose will mar the mask's integrity, and the tears flow faster. I restart twice more before I reach twenty. Finally, the mask comes off, and I weep freely and breathe deeply. I glance at myself in the mirror:

my red, puffy eyes; my face indented from twelve hours a day in this mask. My raw skin. I splash water on my face. Then I wipe my eyes, return my mask to my face and rejoin my colleagues. We continue making our rounds. We wait.

---

**SIMONE BLASER** is an infectious disease physician and scientist at Yale University. Before turning to medicine, she worked in book publishing, where she helped develop *When Breath Becomes Air* with the late Paul Kalanithi. Her narrative medicine prose has appeared in *Clinical Infectious Diseases* and *Clinical Correlations*; her poetry is in *New York City Haiku*.

# Where Are You, Mary Oliver?

KATHARINE LAWRENCE

When I was young, you showed me the river
behind my house.
Not for what it was—
a small, thready thing
moving from the old pump house through tall grasses and
skunk cabbage, white-striped and green and pungent,
disappearing into light-dappled forest
—but for what it might be.
Arrowheads emerged, and frogs,
as cool earth swirled to my ankles
the river plumbed my body, the fields swept on behind
and afternoon dragonflies surveyed their territory.

Where are you, Mary Oliver?
It has been so long since we touched the world,
and all around us is plague.
It's hard to hear your voice on the empty streets, old pavement,
the hospital ward.

I miss the earthworms.

I'm looking to the tree buds
to give a sign that better things are emerging.

I put my ear to the ground
but all I hear are sirens.

---

**KATHARINE LAWRENCE** received her medical degree from Herbert Wertheim College of Medicine at Florida International University and completed a residency in internal medicine and primary care at NYU Grossman School of Medicine, where she is an assistant professor in population health. She is also a teaching attending and hospitalist at the Margaret Cochran Corbin VA Campus in Manhattan. Her clinical and research work advances digital health technologies to improve care delivery and experiences for patients and clinicians. During the COVID-19 pandemic, Lawrence provided direct care to hundreds of New York City veterans and civilians.

SHORT STORY

# Resuscitation

DALY WALKER

Dr. Slater Knotts walked through the emergency room of the hospital where he was head of the pulmonary disease department. He was wrestling with what was best for Amato Bertini, his COVID-19 patient who was critically ill in the ICU. Everywhere he looked he saw people sick with the coronavirus struggling to breathe, being placed on ventilators, or getting CPR. Slater shook his head in disbelief. It was a war zone. Never in his fifteen years of practice had he seen anything close to the suffering this pandemic was causing, not even the AIDS epidemic when he was in training.

At Slater's side was Megan, a tall first-year internal medicine resident who was taking her rotation on Slater's service. She had been at Notre Dame, and became a Rhodes Scholar. Slater considered her to be one of the brightest residents he had trained. But he thought her headstrong and somewhat arrogant. Dressed in personal protective equipment—N95 masks, face shields, gowns, and boots made of PVC—they looked like two astronauts in a space capsule. From the ER, they went to ICU, where an orderly passed them wheeling a gurney that carried a body covered with a sheet.

In a cubicle near the nurses' station, Slater peered down at Mr. Bertini. He removed the semi-comatose man's mask to get a good look at him. A gray stubble of beard sprouted on his chin. His dark hair was oily and matted, his eyes were closed. When he sucked in a breath, his lips pursed, and his skin bore the blue-gray hue of oxygen deprivation. Slater pressed his stethoscope to Mr. Bertini's chest. Each breath he heard was a bubbly heave, a heavy load lifted and dropped. Slater turned to Megan.

"Does he have family?" he asked.

"A son they can't locate," Megan said.

Slater tried to imagine what it must be like to be alone and drowning in your own secretions—the terror, the utter loneliness.

"What are you going to do?" Megan asked.

For a moment, Slater questioned himself. Does his life have meaning? Should we let nature take its course? Or should we save him and commit him to what might be a life of suffering? Mr. Bertini gasped for air and moaned.

"Easy now," Slater said. "We're going to take care of you." He turned to Megan. "He's miserable. We need to make him comfortable. Morphine or a respirator? Those are the choices."

"There's a 'Do Not Resuscitate' order in his chart," Megan said. "You know, he has cancer of the prostate with bony metastasis."

"Prostate cancer won't kill him. The corona infection is benign," Slater said. "We're his caretaker. Even though he's old, we should treat him the way a caring mother would treat her child."

Megan narrowed her eyes and scowled. "He's an adult, not a child." Slater could feel himself getting impatient with her.

"Didn't they teach you the Vatican Declaration on Euthanasia at Notre Dame?"

"No. Why?"

"It says those in the medical profession must not end a life either by a willful act or by withholding care."

"I don't agree with everything the Church says."

"Your concerns are legitimate, Megan. But trust me, the right thing to do is to put Mr. Bertini on a ventilator."

"The hospital is about to run out of ventilators," Megan said. "What if a young person needs one and none are available?"

Her contrariness seemed disrespectful. Slater didn't like being challenged by someone just out of medical school.

"There's an ethics committee to deal with that." Slater looked directly at her. "Our job is to take care of Mr. Bertini."

Megan lowered her eyes and shook her head. Slater stepped out of the cubicle and hurried to the nurses' station. Marlene, the charge nurse, was at the desk.

"What do you need, Dr. K?" she said.

"A ventilator, Marly, and the stuff to intubate Mr. Bertini."

"You sure?"

"That's my decision."

Marlene picked up the phone and started to dial. "Make it stat," he said. "Mr. Bertini is in trouble."

Slater knew the intubation would spray the patient's respiratory droplets on him, and in spite of the protective gear he wore, put him at risk of being infected with the virus. For a moment, he thought of his two children—Ed, age seven and Sue, age five—and his wife, Julie, whose asthma made her precarious. The last thing he wanted was to bring the virus home to them.

He worried that his mask would leak or that his gloves wouldn't protect him. But he put those concerns aside and went back to Bertini.

Soon a lanky inhalation therapist wheeled a ventilator into the cubicle. Marlene appeared behind him carrying a laryngoscope and a plastic endotracheal tube on a towel-covered tray. Slater turned to Megan and pointed toward the scope.

"You do the intubation," he said.

"No, thank you," she said coldly.

"I'll guide you through it."

"I prefer that you do it."

Slater frowned and stepped to the head of the bed. He inserted the blade of the laryngoscope into Bertini's mouth. Slowly, with practiced ease, he exposed V-shaped vocal cords and, beyond, the dark, hollow trachea. He held out his gloved hand, and the therapist placed the tube into it. Slater quickly slid it through the vocal cords and into the trachea.

Bertini's cough made Slater grimace. He blew up the balloon

that held the tube in place. The therapist connected it to the ventilator and switched on the machine. Its bellows swished and sighed. With his stethoscope, Slater listened to Bertini's chest.

"Both lungs are aerated," he said.

Slater stripped off his rubber gloves and dropped them in a waste container. For a moment, he looked down at Mr. Bertini, watching his chest rise and fall like a pendulum that swung in perfect rhythm. Slater turned to Megan.

"As a physician" he said, "there's a fundamental of medicine you need to remember.

"What's that?"

"Death is the enemy. Life is sacred."

Beneath her face shield, her cheeks reddened.

"Patient autonomy is the most sacred thing in medicine," she said.

"I don't believe that's always the case," he said. "When you've been in practice a while, you will come to understand that."

Megan shrugged, then turned and walked away.

On his way home, Slater drove through the rain. The silent, empty streets and unlit shops conveyed an aura of apocalypse. The drops that splattered his windshield reminded him of contaminated droplets spewing from Mr. Bertini's lungs. The car's wipers slapped side to side. Slater had read *The Plague*, by Camus, and he felt like Dr. Rieux traveling through his stricken city, finding it hard to believe that pestilence had crashed down on its people. He came to Shoofly, a chic bar and restaurant. Through a water-speckled window, he could see young people laughing and drinking, crowded together without masks. Their gaiety and disregard for the virus angered Slater. Don't they care about others? He blamed them for him not being able to hug his children or sleep with his wife. He blamed them for Mr. Bertini's illness. He wished they could see his patient and know what fighting for your life is like.

Slater pulled into the driveway of his house and parked in front of the garage. He clicked an automatic opener. The door rattled up revealing his isolation quarters. An old oriental rug covered the cement floor. There was an inflatable bed and a beanbag chair. Julie had covered a small table with a red-and-white checkered cloth. A bottle of Pinot Grigio was chilling in an ice bucket. Slater entered the garage and lowered the door. He stripped off his clothes, and with a towel around his waist went into the house.

"I'm home!" he called.

"I'm giving baths," Julie said from upstairs.

In the laundry room, Slater deposited his clothes in the washing machine and started the cycle. Being careful not touch anything, he went to the downstairs bathroom, where he stepped into a shower with water as hot as he could stand it. He soaped himself from head to toe. For a while, he stood in the steam and let hot water needle his skin. He felt contaminated and drained of energy. His sick patients haunted him. All he wanted was to put the hospital out of his mind, to eat and go to sleep.

Slater went to the inflatable bed, where he lay in the dark feeling sad and totally alone. He was weary of his work, weary of his devotion to his patients. What he craved was the love of his family. A cricket trapped in the garage chirped continuously. Slater thought of the unfairness of the world.

"Goddamn virus," he said.

Two weeks later, it was dark when Slater walked from his car to the hospital. Megan had moved on to an oncology rotation at the cancer hospital. Slater was glad to have her gone, but at the same time he felt he had somehow failed to mentor her properly. Mr. Bertini was still on the ventilator, and Slater was thinking that if the man wasn't able to come off the machine, he would have to do a tracheotomy. He knew a trach was a super-spreading procedure that aerosolized the virus and sprayed droplets on the doctor performing it. The thought of taking the virus home terrified Slater. He prayed he wouldn't have to trach Mr. Bertini.

At the ICU nurses' station, he reviewed Bertini's medical record on a computer screen.

When he saw that the patient no longer required high levels of oxygen, and was tolerating long periods of time off the ventilator, Slater managed a smile. For a moment, he sat thinking. Then he stood up and walked to Mr. Bertini's bedside. The endotracheal tube protruded from his patient's mouth.

"Amato," he said, "if you can hear me, raise your hand."

Mr. Bertini's hand rose from the bed and he opened his eyes.

"Well, hello there." Slater placed his hand on Mr. Bertini's shoulder. "I'm going to let you breathe on your own."

Mr. Bertini nodded his head.

"Just relax and breathe." Slater disconnected the tube from the ventilator and switched off the machine. "That's all you have to do. Breathing is your sole purpose in life right now."

For a long while, he watched Mr. Bertini, noting the excursions of his chest and the color of his skin. He studied the vital signs that scrolled across the screen of the monitor above the bed.

"In and out. Deep breaths. You're doing great, man. I'm going to get that tube out of your throat."

Mr. Bertini made a thumb's-up gesture. Slater summoned Marlene to the cubicle's door and told her he was going to extubate Mr. Bertini.

"Praise the Lord," she said.

She handed Slater a big plastic syringe, which he used to suck the air from the cuff that held the tube in place. Carefully, he slid it from Amato's throat. Mr. Bertini sputtered and coughed. Slater stepped back from the bed to try to avoid contamination.

"Who . . . ?" Amato growled. His voice was husky. He cleared his throat. "Who are you?"

"Your doctor," Slater said.

"Did you put me on that goddamn machine?"

Slater nodded his head. "Yeah, I did."

Amato cleared his throat again "You put me through hell!"

"I'm very sorry for what you've been through."

"Don't be sorry." A slight smile came to Amato's face. "Thank you, Doc." Slater's throat tightened and beneath his face shield his eyes glistened. He wished Megan were here to observe. There was much to be learned at the bedside.

Whenever a COVID patient came off a ventilator, a song was played on the hospital's loudspeaker system. When Slater heard "Every Breath You Take," he smiled. But then the music was interrupted by the sound of a siren, and the red light of an ambulance flashed through the cubicle's window. Soon Slater's pager beeped. He took in a big breath and braced himself for whatever might come next.

---

**DALY WALKER** is a retired surgeon and a fiction editor for *Intima*. His fiction has appeared in *The Sewanee Review, The Louisville Review, The Southampton Review,* the *Catamaran Literary Reader, The Saturday Evening Post,* and *The Atlantic*. His work has been short-listed for the Best American Short Stories, a Pushcart Prize, and an O'Henry Award. He is the author of two collections of stories, *Surgeon Stories* and *The Doctor's Dilemma*. He divides his time between Boca Grande, Florida, and Quechee, Vermont, and teaches a fiction workshop at Dartmouth College in the summer.

ESSAY

# Curveballs

KAITLYN REASONER

As a child, my father would take me to Minnesota Twins baseball games at the Hubert H. Humphrey Metrodome stadium in downtown Minneapolis. As a special treat, sometimes he would buy me a paper scorecard. Always detail-oriented and slightly neurotic, I loved the precision of keeping a scorecard. I would carefully record the 6-4-3 double play or delineate whether a strikeout was a "K" or a "backward K." I don't remember much about entering the stadium. But I have vivid memories of exiting the positively pressurized ballpark, when the push and pull doors would be unlocked to allow the large crowd to exit the stadium more easily and quickly. The pressurized stadium doors would whoosh me out of the Metrodome and into the night summer air to join throngs of fans outside the stadium.

Now, nearly two decades later, I was entering and exiting through pressurized doors in a completely different scenario, in the confines of the hospitals where I worked. Entering the negative pressure of a room or hallway of COVID-19 patients had a similar sensation, but it was not invigorating. It was not exhilarating to know I was walking directly into contaminated air. In preparation, I donned an N95 mask and pinched it carefully around my nose. I wrapped myself in a paper or plastic disposable gown and pulled gloves onto my hands. I put on either safety glasses or a face shield for eye protection. Once this was all in place, I would step into the negative-pressure area.

The Metrodome roof was bright white, puffed up like a marshmallow by the positive-pressure air. With the stadium lights reflecting off the white roof, it always felt intensely bright and almost glaring. In contrast, the rooms of the COVID-19 patients seemed dim and gray. I'm still not sure how much was physical darkness and how much was emotional despair. It turns out that hope can escape even a negative-pressure room. The Metrodome was always loud and lively, with exuberant fans, a booming public address announcer, and a blaring sound system. The COVID-19 rooms were so quiet, often with only the rhythmic whoosh of the BiPAP or ventilator, or the whir of a CRRT machine. The patients lay there alone, typically with no families around.

There were no baseball scorecards in this negative-pressure world. There was only The List. Every day we would "run The List," typically multiple times a day. But in reality, The List ran us. The List held physical reminders of what needed to be accomplished in that particular shift. In the ICU during that time, The List might have various ventilator settings scrawled on it, next to the morning labs and the typical lengthy checklists of to-do items. The List could be used to keep track of which COVID-19 patients' family members I'd managed to update that day. The List could be used to write down the time of death so you'd enter it correctly in the electronic medical record.

If I learned the game of baseball in the positive-pressure world of the Metrodome, then I learned how to be a doctor in the negative-pressure world of the pandemic. I graduated from medical school in the spring of 2020, so I've only ever practiced as a physician in the era of a pandemic. I learned to troubleshoot refractory hypoxia, because it seemed everyone was hypoxic. I learned to stay awake for twenty-eight hours straight and still talk coherently on morning rounds. I learned to break bad news and to have difficult conversations with families, how to gently but directly tell them things were not going well. There was so much bad news. I knelt on the hard floor of the ICU late at night so I could be at a family member's level while I told them how their loved one's organs were failing. I sat quietly in a conference room with a patient's family member to tell them their loved one was dead. I called the medical examiner to report the deaths from a communicable disease.

I appreciate the order and structure of baseball—the crisp infield lines, the precision of a perfectly localized curveball, and how there's a rule for everything. In the Metrodome, there were even rules about what to do if the baseball struck the upper catwalks along the inflated roof.

Medicine certainly has its moments of order and precision, like interpreting an arterial blood gas or calculating a bicarbonate deficit or visualizing your wire inside the internal jugular vein while placing an ultrasound guided central line. But there are countless scenarios with seemingly no rules, that no one can prepare you or train you for, that seem impossible to ever learn or become accustomed to doing. No one can prepare you for pronouncing a proned patient dead. Sometimes, we would prone the COVID-19 patients who had refractory hypoxia, often as a last-ditch effort when we couldn't keep their oxygen saturations up with any other tactics. One of my patients died like that; rotating her to a supine position would likely have hastened her already rapidly approaching death. I struggled to place my stethoscope under her body—literally dead weight—to listen for the absence of heart sounds as part of my death exam.

There is no calculation for how to respond when a family member berates you over the phone when you're just calling to give them an update on their critically ill father who would later die from COVID-19. You'll try to keep your voice even and calm, but you'll feel angry and sad and mostly exhausted. The medical school radiology elective doesn't prepare you for how to show a chest X-ray over a video call to your patient's curious and caring family. There are no guidelines for what to say to the young woman whose fiancé died from COVID-19 and other medical complications. She was a thin wisp of a girl with dark hair, almost ethereal. I pronounced him dead and then she looked at me and said, "We were supposed to get married!" What can you even say to that? No amount of IT training can prepare you for what it feels like to host a Zoom call on your cell phone so that a family can say goodbye to their dying loved one in the middle of the night. There is no protocol for how to blink back tears without touching your eyes and contaminating yourself. The infection prevention guidelines may mandate usage of an isolation stethoscope in rooms under contact precautions. But for the death exams, I tried to use my real stethoscope for that final auscultation—this time for the absence of heart sounds—instead of the flimsy plastic isolation stethoscopes. I felt my patients deserved that courtesy even if it meant I had to take extra time to clean it afterward.

The Metrodome is gone now; I've moved away, and the Minnesota Twins have a new stadium. And the COVID-19 rooms and hallways are gone now too. Sometimes I worry that we'll forget; that we have already forgotten. But it was never the physical spaces, was it? It was never the positive or the negative pressure. It was always the people that shared those spaces with us. I cherish my memories with my dad in the positive-pressure Metrodome. And I remember my colleagues who worked so hard with me in the pandemic. And the negative pressure could not and never will extinguish the memories of the COVID-19 patients. Many of them never made it home. The COVID-19 wards may be closed but the memories of these patients will live on in their loved ones and in those of us entrusted to care for them in that negative-pressure world.

---

**KAITLYN REASONER** is an assistant professor of medicine in the division of infectious diseases at Vanderbilt University Medical

Center in Nashville. Her clinical and research interests are orthopedic infections and antimicrobial stewardship. She is a graduate of Berea College and Vanderbilt University School of Medicine. In her free time, she enjoys hiking, reading, and spending time with her one-eyed cat, Thistle.

# 7

# DEATH SENTENCES

*Feeling Mortal*

# Teatime

### CATHERINE READ

You will learn to greet death like a friend
Ask why he is so intent on taking you now
Let him pull up a chair
He will be shocked you are not afraid of him
   ruining the upholstery

Start to reminisce
Remind him of the time he came for your mother
How she fought him off with chemo and a scalpel
He will mention he was always impressed by her fire

He will still be uncomfortable in your living room
So tell death that if it makes him that nervous
He can kick off his shoes
But this carpet has known more dirt than a gossip
So she's not surprised by anything

He still won't be ready to keep the conversation going
So ask death about the car crash, if he was really there or not
Because your mother and the police swear he was so close
But you never felt like he was even in walking distance

Let him ask you why you are not afraid of him
Death is used to being too taboo
Offer him tea
Tell him he's been in the room with you for too long
   for you fear him anymore

He is more like an acquaintance than an event these days
Five years of passing in the hallways of the hospital
In the midnights you spent with patients who were awake
   and sputtering

In the days you almost fell asleep while driving home
Death was always a gentleman to you
Never came for you before you were ready
But was always nearby in case you needed him

Ask if he wants cream and sugar for the tea
Tell him you trust him now
That he won't force you into anything
He will start to lace up his sneakers again
Tell him you find something poetic in him
Let him laugh

It will feel hollow, will rattle in your chest like the bell tower
  of an empty church
Death will remind you he is not a metaphor, he is all too real
He will tell you your tea was a little strong
Laugh
Tell him his presence has made you fierce
He will tell you that you already were

Don't get up, he knows to close the door on the way out
Ask when he will be back and let the lock click in reply
Smile to yourself
Now, at least, you know what his voice sounds like

**CATHERINE READ** is a surgical resident in Greenville, North Carolina, where she lives with her husband and two boys. Between work, playground trips, and post-call naps, she writes to process the beauty and difficulty of working in medicine.

# Omens

### RYAN BOYLAND

A moth flits around the room,
favoring the exam light, shining
as it is, useless, aimed at the wall.
"That's a bad omen," the nurse says.

I'm not superstitious. I'll call a night quiet
without hesitation. Crip walk on cracks
all the way from the hospital to the parking garage,
mother's back be damned. But something

about her voice ties a thin string of doubt
around my heart. The moth lazily crosses my face,
unbothered. "I think that's a bad omen," she says,
again, and the knot grows tighter.

A man who was speaking to me an hour ago,
who had strong feelings about the temperature
in his room, who was telling me how
he had too many drinks—that's why he was dizzy,

that's why he hit his head, that all this fuss
was for nothing—clung now to life
with every lurching respiration. Breathing tube
in his throat, crusting vomit cornering his mouth,

blood spilling from his right ear.
When I leave the hospital, his husband is
at bedside, stroking his hand, ignoring the blood,
ignoring the faint smell of bleach, a kind of cleanliness

that makes my skin crawl. The artificial,
encroaching on the pure. When I get home,
I lie in bed, spending the next hour checking his
labs on my phone, scrolling, because

while I am awake, he is still alive.
The next morning, I avoid every crack.
A family of moths silently orbit the light
in the stairwell. The knot is so tight I can't breathe.

I walk by his room and see the blood
is gone. The linens are fresh.
His bed is empty

---

**RYAN BOYLAND** is a Pushcart Prize–nominated writer, a wanderer, a doctor, and an amateur astronomer based in Denver, Colorado.

Boyland and his work have been featured on Button Poetry, as well as in *Rattle*, *Omaha Magazine*, *Retrograde Review*, and the *Cookout Literary Journal*. Recordings and performances can be found on YouTube and TikTok. Read more about his work at ryanboyland.com.

SHORT STORY

# Cause of Death

## YU LI

THE MORGUE WAS a nice place to be on a chilly Saturday morning.

I started from the left shoulder of the body, and then the right shoulder. Cutting down to the center point in between two nipples, and a straight line down the abdomen through the belly button. After six years of being an autopsy technician, this work was now routine. The resistance of human skin against the knife held by my hand felt safe and secure.

My patient—we still called them "patients" and the autopsy a "service" even though they were dead—was a twenty-four-year-old male who had passed away yesterday evening in the hospital from respiratory failure.

Respiratory failure was largely an uninformative diagnosis for the cause of death. The patient was a bag of bones. Multiple cancers had over years consumed his young flesh, and finally came a day when he was left with nothing to live on.

I did know a lot about death. Living, instead, was something I was never good at. The nightmares had been bothering me every night, to the point that I always woke up soaking wet with an unbearable nausea.

My best friend Roy walked in. He was fully scrubbed and gowned like a Thai coconut rice dessert wrapped in banana leaves—the signature look of a first-year pathology resident.

"Hey, Tina," he murmured shyly, barely audible with the

ventilator roaring behind.

"Dr. Roy Kovach!" I exclaimed. "What a surprise! Come get me some towels."

Roy blushed predictably because I called him doctor. He opened his mouth a couple of times, trying so hard to find a topic for small talk that he seemed to approach an acute respiratory failure.

Turning back to the autopsy, I examined the patient. Now the skin was divided into a nice symmetrical Y-shape. I worked from the tip of the top triangle and carefully separated the skin from the chest wall, all the way up to the throat. Thin streams of blood emerged, though not too aggressively because the body had been cooled overnight in the fridge. I tucked several towels under the patient's arms so the blood wouldn't contaminate the floor.

Roy stood quietly as I worked, and handled tools like a dedicated operating room nurse.

Most residents would leave the lab when technicians were doing the dirty work, but Roy somehow liked staying around.

He was truly the sweetest human being that I knew of.

How can someone like Roy decide to be a doctor, I wonder. He was not a great communicator. The PhD years were the best time of his life, and then came the clinical rotation that almost ruined his career and resulted in one round of unsuccessful attempts to match into any surgery program. Finally, he was pushed to us at a lower-mid-tier hospital department of pathology, despite his numerous publications and impressive test scores. Even over here, he was not good at talking to fellow residents and attendings. How had he, upon first stepping into the world of medicine, expected patients to possibly appreciate his enormous empathy and warmth if he could not even advocate for or defend himself?

But he cared, I knew.

I tied and snipped the carotid arteries on both sides, reached to the larynx and dissected it from the top of the thyroid cartilage located deep in the neck. The patient's glassy, dead brown eyes, half-open from the external examination I did earlier, met mine. I straightened up and looked at his face. He seemed to have been a joyful young man. Yet now he was pale, thin, and dry, with a faint smile fixed on the corners of his lifeless mouth. The family wouldn't want to see blood on his face and hands when they said the final goodbye. I sighed and grabbed another towel to cover his face.

"So, how was your Friday night?" I asked while quickly shearing off the other two pieces of skin on the side.

Roy smiled with a hint of excitement. "Not bad. I went back to the research building thinking about my project. You know, that one on triple-negative breast cancer. There can be a new way of experiment design, if a combination of immune markers does not necessarily bring the same prediction power as the individual biomarkers do. When we talk about PD-L1, and CD163, and FOXP3 . . ."

He saw me looking at him with amazement. His voice suddenly faded away as if he had just realized what he was talking about—and that a technician, like me, probably would not appreciate the choices of biomarkers nor want to pleasantly discuss the study design with an MD/PhD. He blushed even harder than when he'd come in.

Roy murmured that he'd help, and he quickly grabbed the rib cutter to hide his embarrassment, even though there was nothing to be embarrassed about.

"That's so great, Roy. You'll make some important findings." I smiled at him. Poor Roy. Someone spending his Friday night thinking about biomarkers might not have a much better life than mine. How had I spent my Friday night? Right, I couldn't eat half of my food—the microwaved frozen spaghetti dinner somehow made me feel sick. Then the nightmares. I'd felt almost relieved this morning when I was paged about a new case.

The rib cutter looked a lot like a pruning lopper for gardening, with long handles and curved blades. We used it to remove the chest plate. Roy was not necessarily strong, but he still operated it much more easily than I usually did. I always needed to really push my body weight onto the cutter when dealing with the especially hard first rib.

"Did I ever tell you . . ." I began, "you always make me think about my baby brother."

When we were kids, he'd been the one running in the front, exploring everything with an intense curiosity and explaining them to me in such a serious manner. I'd been the big sister following him and protecting him from behind. We had both believed he'd make a great scientist.

The bones cracked with a strange crispy sound, maybe because the patient had long been osteoporotic. For a while, that was the only sound in the room. Then I heard Roy whisper, "He's very lucky to have a sister like you."

Holding up a rib cutter, we could easily resemble a scene from any horror movie. Things got a lot dirtier in pathology compared to, say, fancy surgery. We did not bother to keep the incision small, the blood loss controlled, nor the scene sterile. What's gone was gone. I sometimes wondered if there were souls floating by the ceiling. They had to be scared as hell watching their bodies undergoing this whole process of dissection.

Roy and I both held our breaths as he flipped the chest plate up.

Cancer. White lumps of poorly differentiated tissues clinging on the inner side of his chest plate, his pericardium—the membrane that wrapped the heart—his lungs, and his diaphragm. I cut into his abdomen and with a small amount of ascites, more cancer was revealed.

The liver was hardly its original organ anymore. A sizable ball of hardened white-yellow overgrown malignant cells had squeezed the normal tissue to one side. A gray-black color appeared on a lengthy section of his necrotic small bowel.

Holy Mother of God. I wondered how he had lived and breathed and eaten with this broken body in the past twenty-something years. When he had walked along the street, heading to his endless hospital visits, had anyone passing by ever realized how broken he was inside and how close to death he'd been?

I clamped the bowels and collected them in a separate tray. Roy watched me doing this less pleasant part of my job.

"How have you been?" His calm voice above me asked. "You look, hmm, exhausted. I have been worried."

"Exhausted" was a euphemism. I had not looked into a mirror for a while, but I knew I was not too different from the saggy, worn-out sofa back in the autopsy office—though it was pleasant to know Roy was worried about me.

"It's been hard." I clamped the lower end of rectum and took out the last part of colon. "You don't understand, Roy, I've been having these horrible dreams, like . . ."

I paused. I suddenly realized I did not actually remember any of the dreams. Except for the enormous sadness they flooded me with. What the hell were they?

"Whatever." I gave up searching for those lost dreams, "Let me pull the entire block of organs out and they're all yours. I'll fix those lungs for ya."

I was looking for my knife, buried under the towels, when the lab door swung open. Michael Chou, a second-year pathology resident, walked in, holding the door with his foot and putting on his gloves at the same time.

"Hey, Tina, sorry I'm late, I saw the page, but the baby started puking . . ." He hurried in, tying his gown carelessly.

I offered him a smile. "Absolutely no worries, Michael. I didn't know you were coming today as well."

Michael asked curiously, "Who else is here today?"

The left lung lay in my hands. I lowered my eyes and stared at it. A squishy, fresh, pink lump of tissue, smaller than you would have imagined, because lungs naturally collapse inward once the chest is open. Spots of cancer cell villages were scattered in it. Without looking up I knew Roy was not there anymore. He was gone. He had been gone.

"No one, just me." I answered quietly.

"Hey, Tina, you know what, leave those to me. You look terrible. I wouldn't be surprised if you told me you were just off a thirty-six-hour shift." Michael looked at me carefully and added softly, "I'm sorry we lost Roy. We all are. But we can pull through it together, right?"

Suddenly my eyes were blurred. I did not know what to say. It must be this face shield, I thought, always fogging up.

I made it back to the office on the other side. Unlike what one might imagine, the autopsy office was a warm, cozy room with wooden desks, outdated computers, and one single old, old sofa no one had ever thought to replace.

How could I so easily forget that Roy had died? Following his suicide, a whole wave of mainstream media featured his case of physician burnout. The entire department was flushed with counseling, grief support groups, and an overwhelming amount of good wishes and nice words. All to prevent the next case from happening.

I was confused. Was Roy burned out? And why did none of us ever realize how close to death he'd been? I had watched this quiet young man grow quieter over the last six months of his life, but he had smiled every time he came downstairs and would always give me a hug if we weren't gowned up. The hugs still felt real to me.

He never mentioned a word about his depression, or whatever they said in the news. He occasionally came to sit on the sofa when I was on call, holding his coffee; he said he enjoyed moments like that. But he never asked for help even when I offered to talk. Had he always been deeply broken inside his mind, day after day until he was too weak to fight—until he had nothing to hope for?

Roy ended it all just before Christmas, the night after he had worked late alone to finish up an autopsy report. I checked that case, and there was nothing special about it. An eighty-nine-year-old female who had survived a good forty years after her cardiac transplant. It should have been a case for life, not death.

Later, there was an email sent from the president of the hospital. The beginning of it read, "We are deeply saddened by the tragic death of our extraordinary and beloved resident, Roy Kovach, MD, PhD. Roy was a caring, compassionate young physician-scientist in the first year of the pathology residency program. He was a leader and a dedicated explorer of scientific investigations, driven by a desire to offer hope to those who suffer from deadly diseases."

It sounded largely like a Roy I did not know. Instead, I stared at the word "beloved" for a little while. I had lost my baby brother in a car accident when he was four. It was the same word inscribed on his headstone.

I'd been missing him ever since.

---

**YU LI** is a pediatrician-in-training and an aspiring writer. She grew up in Nanjing, China, and now lives in Pennsylvania. She loves writing on the Amtrak train. Her short stories have appeared in *Eunoia Review* and *100 Word Story*.

SHORT STORY

# No Word

E. E. TOKSU

*Dear Mr. Noah Webster,*

*I was at your New Haven home once; I saw where you compiled the first American dictionary. Here are some beginnings of letters I've penned, none of which you'll see or are finished, except this first and the last. Please consider the source, someone who is thrashing around in many directions for answers.*

*Sincerely, Chris*


Dear Mr. Webster,

Thank you for learning many languages to put together the first American dictionary. Adding words that weren't in British English, like "skunk" and "squash," to your lexicographer's collection was practical on your part. Making other words, like "labor" and "color," easier to spell is also much appreciated. I think you missed an opportunity, though, in that there are words missing you may have found along your language studies path.

Dear Mr. Webster,

If you couldn't manage to think of a word to define parents who lose children when even your family lost a child, not to mention the majority of your peers who did too, how are we supposed to have a chance now when losing one is extremely rare? You learned how many languages to compile your dictionary? Couldn't you have found the one word that would have helped: "Vilomah," a word in Sanskrit, one of the languages you studied, that defines us?

Dear Mr. Webster,

I'm sure you wouldn't have done this if you had known the ramifications. That not having a word or even the existence of a category—in the new world, at least—for the survivors of this type of senseless loss leaves them unlisted, off the map, and nonexistent to the rest who remain at the unnerving celebration that is life. You should know from all the maladies from your era, at a time when parents were advised not to become too close to their children until they were toddling steadily into childhood.

Dear Mr. Webster,

I'm afraid you may be a horse's arse. You didn't find a word for a child who dies young, the counterpart to the parent who lost the child. No word for so many young people who were here but couldn't stay. For the precious and pudgy and precocious littles or the young saplings with beautiful light green leaves with all the promise of far future seasons.

By default, young people who die are thought of and referred to as angels. Mine was much more and much less than an angel. Even at age five, almost a third through his time with us, when his grandmother, pushing him in a swing on a stay in Quebec City, called him *mon ange* to imitate the other mothers there, he answered "What's that!?" When she told him the English translation, "my angel," he answered in between being pushed into the air and falling back down to her, "Boys aren't angels . . . well some are, but I'm not."

You spent far too many years on words that don't count, on the ones we don't have or need or use anymore because he's gone. Even if you had put in a portmanteau that blames us, like "childloser," it would have been at least on the record. We give ourselves names anyway if we don't have one: "loser of children," if you prefer. I would have appreciated something like "childloserville" too, since parents who lose children live in that state for some time. Even if they leave during the day, their broken compass brings them back at night. It can't be because your era put dead children into family paintings as if they were still alive and there, is it? Maybe there's something there, but we don't go there in this era where death is taboo, thanks partly to you.

Dear Mr. Webster,

We didn't get the memo not to get close to our young ones or even not to be in a hurry to name them because it would be too hard if they were to die. Come to think of it, you should have had a word for that warning in the dictionary since that would have at least opened up the door to having a word for children who die. Maybe then we wouldn't be singing to bloated bellies to cross to the little-person-inside-the-big-person barrier before we meet.

Dear Mr. Webster,

You had the only control in the face of parents' helpless hell and you frittered it away, as if you might cause it to happen if you named it. Or maybe you were worried that parents would be vilified if there were a name for their post-loss selves. Also, because you were not a maker-upper of words, you would have had to look even further into Sanskrit than you did. Or to China, where there is a word for parents who lose a child when the parents are elderly, 独, perhaps since that must have been when they really needed their children to take care of them.

"Vilomah" is a Sanskrit word for a parent whose child has died and where "widow" and "widower" come from. Either of these words would have been fine. Grieving parents could have wrapped themselves in the word entirely or jumped recklessly from consonants, over valleys of vowels and to the next steep consonant, or written the label over and over in blank notebooks to address even a pinch of the pain, even though it starts like new again the next day. It would have given us something to hold on to that we could run around and make ourselves dizzy until sick. Could have been nice just to know it was there and if there were other Vilomahs out there holding on to that word too. I would have known who my future role models were and perhaps have been taken under their wing even before the loss, during his illness, although I probably would have been too scared to admit I would be in their shoes.

Perhaps having a word would at least have stopped people from crossing the street instead of having to speak to us without the right words. Would have made it so, even for a second, to those who think they can avoid it in their own lives by avoiding us. Instead of leaving us balancing on one toe on a sharp shard island with no water to swim across. Knowing your child is going to die, down to the year and month, from the brainy doctors, and waiting for it not to be, and then, when he's so sick, for it to be, was like being pregnant with a stiller and stiller newborn. I could have earned all seven letters of that Vilomah vernacular by the time his other sneaker dropped.

But I had no label waiting for me to at least tell me who I could possibly be or why I should stay on a planet that lets its sweetest spin off. That word could have been at least a swinging suspension bridge over the abyss of who I was and who I would be. Instead, I packed up my two-ton brick of sorrow, rage, and guilt, and hit the museum trail to find works of art that looked like me, how I felt. Then I became reacquainted with literary and historical figures who had been in my shoes, starting with *The Testament of Mary*, which gave me permission to destroy the whole world and resurrect it again by pushing past the hardness first.

Dear Mr. Webster,

Not for nothing, but since there's no one hard-edged word and only soft and stuffy euphemisms in your word collection in print, at least let there be many empty pages in the middle of your book where siblings and parents could draw or press mementos of their children. Put them into your book like a do-it-themselves kit. We have someone named Martha Stewart who would be all over that. Such a project may help prepare parents too, each time they see those empty pages, if anything can. At least there'd be a place to go in addition to the grave. In your era you engraved on cemetery headstones that the dead "departed their life." We should also say that nowadays; it gives the sick or the hurt or the murdered more agency, even the sin of human pride before a fall. They walk offstage rather than wait for the curtain to come down.

Dear Mr. Webster,

*I am sorry for your profound loss. There are no words to express my sympathy for your family's loss of your child, who is most certainly the most beautiful angel in heaven watching over you.*

*In sympathy,*

*Chris*

---

**E. E. TOKSU** is a patient advocate in New York City. She holds an MS degree in narrative medicine from Columbia University.

ESSAY

# The Boxer

ANIQA AZIM

I DON'T TELL my husband, but at night I think about Tom. When I met Tom, he was already bed-bound and translucent. His skin was placed on bone like loosely laid gift wrap.

His eyes were transfixed upon a spot on the ceiling, half closed, like he was asleep. At first, we were waiting for a liver transplant.

For three days, I pumped laxatives into him and waited for him to tell me all the stories his son had already shared:

About Tom, the boxer, from a line of boxers. Tom, the fighter, undefeated, roaming around the world, showing off his courage. Tom, the father, distant, tough, but always proud of his boy.

We just need to get him to poop out all the toxins from his blood, I explained to his son, with confidence.

After three days, I sent Tom to the ICU for dialysis, to help him circulate the toxins out of his blood.

It's where he needs to be, I asserted, while I briskly paged the ICU fellow downstairs, begging them to accept him.

My last page was just: he looks so bad.

On the fourth day, the ICU sent Tom back up to me to die.

The intensivist tried not to be unkind: "Look at him, how could anyone think of trying to do a transplant on this guy, when he might not even make it through the night?"

Tom's wife had told me he had been diagnosed with rheumatoid arthritis the year before, and at first, he didn't think much of the pain and swelling in his joints.

But it turns out the swelling was just a clue that Tom's body was launching an attack on itself.

The last front: the liver.

The victim: Tom.

On the fifth day, I told Tom's son that he was dying. By now he knew the drill. "From toxins in his blood?"

Yes, I affirmed.

The mitochondria are the powerhouse of the cell.

The liver helps clear toxins in the blood. When the liver fails, the kidneys can fail.

The phrases we use to explain that bodies and people are as fragile as paper, as delicate as gift wrap.

Tom's wife didn't come to the hospital that night.

"He had so much machismo," she said. "He wouldn't want me to see him like this."

Sometimes I wish I didn't have to see him like that either.

Or maybe that I didn't see him like the full-faced man he was in the picture by his night table. Young, strong, a boxer without rheumatoid arthritis or a scarred, malfunctioning liver, or toxins in his blood.

Some contrasts are so stark you cannot make sense of one thing in the face of the other.

When I heard Tom had died, I understood it to be a natural progression of his disease. I walked down the hall, sighed, thought, "That was a sad outcome."

I walked into the team room with a cup of burned coffee and a determination to get through the day.

I made fun of a coworker, I browsed around on my phone, aimlessly scrolling.

But—the night before Tom died was the last time I had slept in a month. Now I am awake. I am always awake.

These are hidden battles—for sleep, for health, for a liver—fought in private, fought alone.

When I run, I run miles away from the hospital, but I also run to get away from the hospital. When I cry, I think of Tom and Janice and Hector and all the others, losing and dying, but also free.

Some days, it feels like I am fighting to live.

I hope Tom is in another place, fighting for joy.

---

**ANIQA AZIM** is an internal medicine physician. After completing her training and a year as chief resident at Oregon Health and Science University, Azim moved to University of California, San Francisco, where she is an academic hospitalist interested in medical humanities and medical education. When she isn't reading historical fiction or working, Azim enjoys traveling and hiking with her husband.

ESSAY

# To Pronounce

## THOMAS J. DOYLE

*To pronounce: a transitive verb meaning to declare officially or ceremoniously.*

THE PAGER'S STRIDENT ring shakes you out of sleep. It's 4:30 AM. You call the hospital's fifth floor and hear the nurse's voice—calm, deliberate: "Mrs. S in 5043 passed. Can you come and pronounce her?"

As the covering night doctor, you handle everything—including the death pronouncements of patients whom you have never met. The nurse mentions that Mrs. S died alone, with no one at the bedside.

As the early morning light filters through the hospital, you walk to room 5043. Your steps slow and you pause, then knock quietly. You enter the room to find yourself alone with Mrs. S.

She is in the hospital bed to your right, an immaculately clean cotton blanket tucked fastidiously around her upper arms in a swaddling embrace. She is thin, elderly, and her eyes are closed. Is she peaceful? It is difficult to place her expression. She is drained of color, absent of breath.

The whiteboard on the wall has been updated with the name of Mrs. S's nurse. Under "Today's Plan," the word "COMFORT" is written in black ink, with no scheduled procedures, no specimens to be obtained. Under the heading "Discharge" is written: "TBD." Determined by whom?

The television perched high on the wall facing the bed is tuned to the hospital's "Care TV" channel—slow-moving images of shimmering ponds and forests, with calming, meditative music warbling in the background.

You prepare to verify, to diagnose death. Out of habit, you reach for a radial pulse, her skin already cool to your touch. No radial. No carotid pulse. You rub her sternum. No response.

You note that her pupils are fixed, dilated. You check for any sign of a pulse, any breath for more than a minute, then another minute, then for more time. Why? You always feel a vague paranoia, an anxiety to be absolutely sure of death, beyond any doubt. No final agonal gasp, no cardiac escape rhythm, and no chance she will wake up in the morgue.

You look around the room. There is a lone sympathy card on the side table, no flowers, and almost no other personal items. In that moment, you feel acutely the sensation that comes during such a pronouncement in an empty room—an almost out-of-body experience—tremendously sad.

When family is present there are cries, wails, those who pace in and out of the room in the first moments of mourning. You enter those rooms as physician, but also intruder, into the liminal space between the stillness of death and the suddenly poignant transience of life. You sometimes feel akin to the grim reaper, stethoscope in hand.

With family and friends in the room, the sense of the altered reality of the diagnosis of death takes on a magnified intensity. There is an uncomfortable theater to some of these pronouncements, as you place your stethoscope on the chest of the deceased, listening to silence. The mourners at the bedside observe your every movement, hang intently on your words as you offer condolences.

Once, as you arrive, a daughter of the deceased is literally climbing onto the bed. As you wait quietly in the corner, she clings to the body of her mother, holding in one hand a cell phone to live stream the moments after her mother's passing to a sister in Portugal whose muffled howls of grief echo unnaturally in the room.

Another evening, as you enter a room for a pronouncement, you are unexpectedly welcomed, even beckoned, to join the many people gathered at the bedside of an emaciated man in his mid-sixties who has just died. The mood in the room is paradoxically light.

The TV is off and acoustic guitar music comes from a small CD player in the corner. There is a tray of cookies and snacks and a pot of coffee to sustain the mourners in their vigil. The deceased man was a musician, his friends tell you, and his death was a release from weeks of suffering from terminal cancer. He died quietly, at peace, with no words of love or caring left unsaid.

Mrs. S, on the other hand, had almost no friends or family. Her nurse tells you that the closest relative was a grandniece only peripherally involved in her care. Before you complete the death certificate and prepare to call her grandniece, you read the medical record to see what you can learn about Mrs. S.

Your time in the chart is best spent reading notes from the palliative care nurses. They are rich in family detail about Mrs. S in youth, later life, and her recent fight against cancer. You skip dozens of physician notes, glossing over notes from consultants who signed off days ago.

Mrs. S had successful treatment of localized breast cancer many years before, but then, in her late eighties, the cancer recurred and metastasized. Some notes mention consideration of a final attempt with palliative chemotherapy to salvage a few weeks of life. But her malignancy had overtaken her frail body, and just two days earlier Mrs. S shared in, even directed, the final decision to change her code status to "comfort measures only" and enter hospice care. She remained in the hospital on a morphine drip until you were summoned to pronounce her death.

Some might say that this familiarity with her case is unnecessary. Mrs. S died, and what her family needs is a death pronouncement and signature on her death certificate so the logistics of funeral and burial can begin.

But you know the value of familiarity with the life of the deceased you are asked to pronounce. You recall uncomfortably a death many years ago in the middle of the night during a busy shift. You had to squeeze in a pronouncement between care of a patient needing transfer to the ICU and an urgent admission in the ER. You knew only the patient's name and that she died in hospice care in the hospital. As you left the room you were pursued into the hallway by the patient's daughter, tears streaming down, with a question about her deceased mother's final days. You were uninformed, unable to answer in a way that could comfort.

It may sound strange, but after many years of medical practice and hundreds of inpatient death pronouncements, you have acquired a certain skill in this grim duty of medicine. This expertise feels rooted in the most basic tools of medicine. You hope that by pronouncing death with care, respect, and humility, you ease death's burden just a bit for families—and for yourself.

**THOMAS J. DOYLE** graduated from the Warren Alpert School of Medicine at Brown University in 2003 and completed training in general internal medicine at Rhode Island Hospital in 2006. He practices hospital medicine in Massachusetts and Rhode Island. Find more of his work at tjdoyle.com.

# Haglund's Deformity

ELIZABETH LANPHIER

Waking at night
I hold my breath.
I will collect it later,
from a give-a-penny-take-a-penny
dish of air.
If I remember the stars
are not light shining
through holes in a painted black ceiling
like the set of a play, I wonder
where is the seam of the universe?
My stomach gets softer, there is a fresh crease
at the corner of my eye like a no-longer dog-eared page,
and the Haglund's deformity
hardening on my heel has a diagnosable name.
I worry about the hairline fracture on my central incisor
and what would happen if
I had to live forever
without a tooth. A smile's

door off its hinges
that can't be pulled closed.
Skin will become
slack and translucent like
saran wrap removed and then
replaced until it no longer
covers the veins showing through
the back of a hand
that as a kid used to be
stained blue black from the
pens of friends drawing
stars and hearts, now constellations
of sun and liver spots will dot a map
of purple creeks and tributaries
that wind toward the heart
until they one day dry up.
I want to be held
in crepuscular hours
before the drought.

**ELIZABETH LANPHIER** is a philosopher and clinical ethicist. She earned her PhD in philosophy from Vanderbilt University and an MS in narrative medicine from Columbia University, where she is also a lecturer in the certificate program. Lanphier has published poems in *The Examined Life Journal*, as well as scholarship on topics related to feminist philosophy and bioethics, trauma-informed ethics and practice, and narrative methods in health care.

ESSAY

# First Will and Testament

ANNA STACY

The summer I was nineteen, I lived in a small first-floor apartment in Pasadena, on a magnolia-lined street. It was the first apartment I had ever rented. There was no furniture, nothing in the room but a handful of wire hangers, and the air conditioner spewed a hot dust whenever it was on. I found a futon and a fan, and a milk crate to use as a bedside table. My roommate had a large TV in the living room and told me I could use it if I agreed to feed his sourdough starter when he was away. This, I agreed, was a fair arrangement.

The apartment was a few blocks away from the lab where I worked, and the walk there was sublime. I passed flowers in full bloom, a fountain filled to bursting, a pond with turtles basking on the rocks, rows of towering buildings, California-old. And all the while, the sun blazed down and made it shine and shine. Some days, it felt like torture to enter that dark building, to work at the computer in that windowless room with the hum of the refrigerator that stored sections of monkey brains, sliced like deli meat.

Once a week, I'd venture out in the other direction, past the magnolias, past the houses, past the church that looks exactly like a chicken's face, the In-N-Out Burger shrouded in a cloud of weed, the bus stop with the movie poster four years late. The mountains far away would shimmer like a mirage, like something boiling, like a spell. I'd bring along my large tote bag and walk, feeling my skin toast like a soft-shelled nut.

And there, along the strip mall, between the furniture store and the coffee shop, stood the recruiter in a tight black shirt and khaki cargo pants. The sign reading "Army Recruiting Center" was, inappropriately, a navy blue, the letters displayed in a burly stencil font. The recruiter always recognized me. I never caught his name.

"Hey!" he'd call. "Don't you want to travel? Make a difference? Get paid?"

Most days I would walk past without a word. Sometimes I'd offer a tight, polite smile, the way that girls are taught to do, the way that women forget to unlearn. Sometimes I'd ignore him altogether, as if he were a part of the building itself. But sometimes—the lonely days, the days when I really was nineteen—I'd listen to what he had to say with a sarcastic curiosity.

"Don't you want to travel? Make a difference? Get paid?" "Of course," I'd reply. "But I don't want to die." The recruiter would shake his head with a smile. "That doesn't always happen." I'd shake my head right back, then continue on to the grocery store. On my way home, I'd take the bus.

A few months later, in the autumn, I applied to medical school through an Early Assurance Program for undergraduates with significant interests outside of medicine. When I heard about the program, I thought, Hey, that's me! At my interview, the admissions officers talked about how a career in medicine would allow us to heal patients in ways both big and small, to advocate for those who lack a voice. All the loud and exciting parts of being a doctor: make-a-difference, change-the-world. I remember feeling dizzy with all the possibility—the chance to cure, and save, and make people live! It was noble, and it was proud.

I never thought, not even once, that I might die because of it.

In April 2020, in the spring when I was twenty-five, I sat down at my desk early one morning. I had been volunteering at the hospital for a week. In that time, I had heard the break room jokes morph from "When this is over, the bridge of my nose is going to be permanently flat from these damn masks" to "If you take the last muffin, I swear to God I'm writing you out of my will." We all loved joking about our wills—writing them, amending them, burning them, hiding them. I got the sense that others had actually written their wills. I overheard two residents chatting quietly in the Emergency Room, their heads down, their tired eyes just visible behind their face shields. They had their phones out. One said to the other, "Okay, I just sent it to you. If something happens, send that to Mark, okay?"

So, I sat down to write mine.

I had no idea what to include. I didn't have that much stuff. But I had furniture now—a bed frame, not a futon. An air conditioner that worked. A bookshelf full to bursting, titles crammed in sideways and on the diagonal like the tenants of my apartment building. These, I wrote, would go to my roommate, to distribute to our friends as she saw fit. Same with my clothes: whatever people like, whatever's in their size. My brother would get my instruments. And whatever was in my bank account was to be split among my friends to help pay off their student loans, which wasn't much but which I'd hoped would help.

I folded this up—handwritten, as neatly as my almost-doctor handwriting would allow—and put it in an envelope.

Each morning before I set off for the hospital, I would leave the envelope on my desk, as prominently as I could. Just in case my roommate would need to find it. I did this for months.

Shed my scrubs on the landing. Washed my hands until they bled.

Now I am twenty-six, and it is spring again. The bridge of my nose is fine, if sore. My hands are chapped.

My heart is full. That nineteen-year-old had no idea what she was signing up for. I hope that wherever she is, she is well.

---

**ANNA STACY** is a New York–based writer, actor, and emergency physician. Their work has appeared in journals such as *Calyx* and

*Carve*, as well as in the internationally award-winning web series *Dead-Enders*. Stacy is the proud recipient of the Judith and Nathan Kase Humanities in Medicine Prize for their involvement in the arts alongside patient care. Learn more about their work at annastacy.com.

# 8

# THE WONDER YEARS

*Curiosity and Tenderness*

POEM

# Letter to a 93-Year-Old Cadaver Who Died from Multiple Causes

JENNIFER STELLA

I opened your willing body
as an act of love.

The pleasure in dissecting
fascia. Pleasure
in removing clothes.

I never held your hand
ungloved. It was more intimate—your
brittle fingers cradled in my palm, other
hand guiding the scalpel. Probing
nerves or arteries or whatever
loses color.

Reflecting your thoracic cage—not my
saw to your manubrium, not

my cut haphazard-sliced your
lung. Dense, dark. With cartilage
compressed like tears.

Hesitant, macerating muscle, I
glided over your fifth rib, reached
back, twisted my aching wrist up in
inchoate effort to help you
breathe. With child-sized tubes.

The worry when I detached
your heart. Worry when I
spliced your small intestine, removed
your spleen, unsheathed your arms
and legs. Without Anubis-headed jars
or natron linens.

And the staples close to lost
in the louvers of your chest—you
had been opened before. The plastic
mimicking valve. Illicit reconnection.

Stunned by brachial plexus. Triumphant
twinned arch. And your exquisite
heart. Fleur-de-lis aorta. Scalloped edges
of left ventricle fluttered

open. Tendon chords like
butterflies can rupture.

Did you know how beautiful
you were disintegrating.

---

**JENNIFER STELLA** is a writer and doctor. After serving in the Peace Corps, she completed medical school in San Francisco and an MFA in poetry while working as a doctor on Rikers Island. Her writing has appeared in *Calyx*, *Tupelo Quarterly*, *Eleven Eleven*, and *Pharos*. Stella has published two chapbooks, *Your Lapidarium Feels Wrought* and *Letters We're Allowed*. She works with Doctors Without Borders, most recently in Haiti.

ESSAY

# A Shot of Perspective

## JORDANA KRITZER

It was close to 8 am, and we gathered in a circle to receive our first vials. I felt like I was in a movie. So many moments seemed surreal during the past year, like when people started wearing masks to the grocery store, I remember looking at strangers and thinking, "Are we really doing this?" The white medical tents set up outside my hospital during the peak of the pandemic looked like something out of *E.T.* The lockdowns and curfews and endless sirens—it all felt like the script of a Hollywood drama. And now, holding the vial of COVID-19 vaccine in my hand, I felt the camera move in for a close-up.

I had arrived at the Department of Mental Health in Lower Manhattan at 6:30 am. Twenty-five nurses had crowded into a conference room, waiting for their foreheads to be scanned for fever. Once we'd been cleared, the nurse with the clipboard asked for volunteers to give the vaccinations. I raised my hand.

"What are you? It doesn't say on the sheet. RN? LPN?" she asked.

"MD," I muttered, trying not to sound pretentious.

All heads turned to look at me.

"MD?" she whooped. "I don't think I've ever seen an MD here before. Well, I am coming to you if there are any emergencies."

We were told to gather all of our vaccination supplies from a storage room filled with unmarked boxes of needles, syringes, alcohol swabs, Band-Aids, gloves, Lysol spray, gauze, and blank vaccination cards. I had expected to find a box at each vaccination station filled with all the materials I would need for the day. Or at least a list. But then I realized, it's the nurses who put boxes like that together—and that's me today.

I am not new to figuring it out on the fly. I am an emergency medicine doctor—it's practically listed in my job description to be resourceful. I regularly perform surgical procedures on top of sterile-y-draped garbage cans. I have delivered a baby in a stuck elevator and in the back seat of an SUV. But today I was a set of hands, well worn with years of giving injections to patients in distress. I had answered the call to be part of the army of capable hands, a cog in the giant machine designed to pull us out of this pandemic. So I carried what I could find down to the auditorium.

The program manager opened an ordinary, nondescript Coleman cooler and removed the vials. "These are your responsibility," he said. "Every dose is precious and must be accounted for." I looked down at the glass vial pressed against the creases of my palm. The word MODERNA written in red matched its bright red cap. Was this the end of the movie? I thought. Is this the final image that means everything is going to be okay?

"Oh, please let this be the end," I mumbled, almost aloud.

We were told to get to our posts and be ready. My station was on the stage in the auditorium. I double-checked all my supplies and waited.

"Should I begin my eight bars?" a woman in her late seventies crowed as she skipped up the stairs to the stage, her arms extended as if she were to break into song. Her legs found a spryness in this moment that allowed her to float toward me. Her eyes sparkled playfully. "I feel like I'm at an audition."

"Step right up for your golden ticket," I played back. "Have a seat and we'll get this show on the road!"

She sat in the chair, her eyes never leaving mine, tears glistening. "You don't know what this means. I haven't seen anyone in a year. I've been so lonely. My heart has broken so many times. What it will be like to hug my children, my grandchildren. To be in the same room with them, not feel so utterly alone."

I plunged the needle into the vial and drew back her dose. "I can't believe that this is the magic potion," I said. I couldn't help myself. I wanted to soak in this moment as much as she did. I could feel my throat get tight, my own emotion overwhelming my usual defenses.

I thought of the sobs of my patients' families when I called to tell them their loved one was dying from COVID-19. In those moments I had tucked my own feelings away, locked them in the place where I was trained to compartmentalize them, so I could keep doing my job. I specialize in emergency resuscitation, and part of that job has always been end-of-life care, spending someone's final moments with them and their families. But the volume during the peak of the pandemic made for a very full compartment. The desperate requests of my patients' families echoed in my mind.

"Please hold her hand. Tell her I love her. Tell her she is everything to me."

"Tell her I'm sorry. It's my fault. I should have brought her earlier."

"Does he have his glasses? He'll be so scared without his glasses."

"But I just dropped him off! I'm right outside! They won't let me in. Ask him to hold on until I can say goodbye."

"But she's my best friend. I can't live without her."

I blinked back to the present. I really looked at the woman in front of me. And to my surprise, I felt the clasp on that feelings compartment start to open. Her joy was palpable, and instead of noting it as part of my clinical assessment, I felt it. Deeply. I couldn't believe how dangerous and wonderful it felt to allow myself to share in her elation. All of a sudden, I wanted to jump into a pool filled with feelings.

I thought about when I was infected with COVID-19. At the time, we didn't know much about the disease; we had some data from China and Italy, but nothing conclusive. I sent a group message to my ER doctor friends: "Save me a ventilator and watch my teeth when you intubate me—they're real," with a wink emoji, a gallows-humor joke to my friends who, like me, take patients' dentures out before putting a tube down their airway. The text was a joke, and it wasn't.

We were all worried that we would be one of the unlucky few who developed severe COVID-19. There were few if any ventilators left at our hospital. I knew we were all concerned about what we would do if we ran out and a patient needed a "vent," but also, what if they were all gone when *we* needed one?

I thought about how guilty I've felt during this past year. Guilty for the relief I'd feel every time I'd walk through the front door of my warm, beautiful apartment after a difficult shift. I'd see my three young children waiting to hug me as I stripped off my dirty scrubs in the hallway, and I'd think of how many of my patients' families would forever be wishing for them to come through the door.

The woman's masked face became blurry as my own eyes filled with tears. People always ask me—especially this year—if I get emotional witnessing human loss and suffering in my work. I usually say that I leave the emotions to my patients and their families. That it's inappropriate to ask them to shoulder my emotional response on top of having their own. The doctor should take care of the patient, not the other way around. But deep down, I stay behind the wall as a self-protective measure, a shield from the barrage of other people's heartbreak. And until this moment, I hadn't realized how much I've missed out on truly sharing joy with people by protecting and hiding my authentic self.

I don't do Happy Medicine, I thought. The work I do is important, it's fulfilling, it's exciting, but it's not happy. In my busy emergency department, everyone always needs something from me. I always have to decide, even when I'm uncertain. There are too many problems I can't fix. But like so many things, you can only know light if you have been in the dark. And for me, giving a highly effective vaccine during a deadly pandemic comes about as close to pure Happy Medicine as you can get.

I stuck the needle deep in the woman's deltoid muscle, and my thumb easily guided the plunger of the syringe forward. The effort of thousands of scientists, hundreds of thousands of volunteers, and millions of dollars disappeared into her arm in a second. I removed the needle and applied pressure with a bit of gauze.

"It's done!" I cheered.

"That's it?" she asked incredulously.

"Just like that. You're vaccinated!" I placed a Band-Aid over the small hole and handed her the white vaccination card.

"You have received the second shot and completed your vaccination series, congratulations!"

"What do I do now?" she asked.

"Go live your life!"

And all at once, the camera pulls back to view the whole auditorium as the tinkling of instrumental music starts to build. We follow her as she zips up her jacket and walks out into the lobby. She pauses a moment at the door and takes a deep breath. The music swells as she steps out into the bright snowy morning.

---

**JORDANA KRITZER** is a graduate of SUNY Downstate College of Medicine, where she first combined her passions for science and storytelling. After years of directing plays in New York City, she found her way to emergency medicine and completed her training at the Albert Einstein College of Medicine, where she was named the 2015 EM Physician of the Year. Kritzer is now a board-certified assistant professor at Albert Einstein College of Medicine and a member of the Leo M. Davidoff Society for excellence in teaching.

ESSAY

# For the Old Man Buying a Stuffed Giraffe

BEN GOLDENBERG

My career in medicine is always introducing me to new emotional experiences, but nothing will ever make me feel the way I do when I walk into a hospital gift shop. It's like stepping through an interdimensional portal; the frenetic, anxious atmosphere of the hospital gives way to the anodyne hum of small-stakes commerce so seamlessly it's almost jarring. When I enter the gift shop, I'm suddenly in a world where I never have to hear bed alarms or overhead code blue announcements—only the soft rock offerings of 93.9 Lite FM Chicago. Tubes of every Pringles flavor climb the walls like ivy and nobody's talking about vital signs. I can take in a deep, carefree breath of air that smells like greeting cards and tell myself that in this moment there are no major medical decisions to be made. I'm just a guy on a little errand.

Anyway, I'm in the gift shop when I see you. We met briefly last year when you were here with your wife, who at the time was admitted for fever after chemotherapy decimated her white blood cell count. I came to see her as the infectious diseases consultant, and while I don't remember specifics about her case, I remember how thoroughly the room was adorned—get-well cards, flowers, stuffed animals, matching coffee mugs with fading images of Looney Tunes characters, an old souvenir-framed photo of your kids on a roller coaster that doesn't exist anymore.

I remember your satisfied smile as you looked at me and my team members admiring all the knickknacks and tchotchkes that you had lovingly arranged just so. We all just stood there for a while, thinking about our own knickknacks and tchotchkes and the people they remind us of. For a moment, you made everyone in that beige-walled hospital room feel like they were somewhere else. Somewhere better.

Now, months later, she's back in the hospital and you're back in the gift shop's stuffed animal section. I see you holding a bear in one hand and a giraffe in the other. You're alternately lifting each of them up and down as high as your arthritis will allow, slowly and deliberately, like a balance scale weighing gold bullion. I can imagine the gears turning in your head as you wonder which one she'll like more. Which one will better complement the others in the cotton-filled menagerie she's accumulated over the last few months? Which one is more likely to make the next chemo treatment a little more palatable?

I try not to think about the possibility that no matter which animal you choose, she might not recognize it, given the way her cognition and alertness have become more sporadic with each cycle. Will she even be awake enough today to notice a new gift, to notice you? Maybe not, you think, but you decide on the giraffe and shuffle over to the register because at the end of the day it's a gift and it's from you and that's what matters. This is the hospital gift shop, after all, where hope springs eternal and we can temporarily forget about all the suffering this building was constructed to hold. I catch you picking up a few other items, but I get distracted by the radio's smooth transition from "Keep on Loving You" into "The Boys of Summer," and before I know it, you're out the door.

Just before the door closes, though, I can see that you're carrying a trio of Mylar balloons, and they're the shiniest Mylar balloons I've ever seen in my life. And maybe I'm still imagining things but as you walk further down the hallway, I swear I can already hear the hiss of air leaking out of them.

**BEN GOLDENBERG** is a doctor who specializes in infectious diseases. He lives in Chicago.

# A Tale of Three Breasts

## CAROL SCOTT-CONNER

Three of us sit facing a nice young woman who is finishing her general surgery residency and now has applied for our breast surgery fellowship. I'm a breast cancer surgeon. To my right is my colleague from radiation oncology, and to my left, a plastic surgeon who specializes in complex reconstructions after cancer surgery. The young woman is the first applicant we will interview during a highly choreographed morning leading up to the Match, when residents are matched with programs.

This candidate is doing quite well. She answers all of our questions with practiced fluency, and asks a few appropriate but not too revealing questions of her own. She does so well that we run out of questions before we run out of time.

My plastic surgery colleague passes a sheet of paper and a pen across to our candidate and says, "Draw a breast."

"What?"

"Draw a breast! Front and side views. Draw a breast."

Suddenly she looks like a frightened kid. She stares at the paper and pen as if she's never seen either before in her life, then hesitantly reaches out and takes them. For the first time during the interview, she's dumbstruck. All of her attention is focused on the plastic surgeon.

The radiation oncologist and I watch with interest. Neither of us would have thought to ask this.

The kid slowly draws a pair of circles and says, "This is how we draw them? In clinic? To explain to the patients?" The administrative assistant knocks on the door—it's time for this applicant to leave and the next to enter. We ignore the knock.

"Fine," says the plastic surgeon, although it really doesn't look fine to me. Breasts aren't circular, they actually have a tail of tissue that extends up and out toward the shoulder. The plastic surgeon goes on, "Now draw a side view."

The kid draws a half-moon. It could be a breast, but it could also be half of a tomato, the waning half-moon at midnight, or a brimless baseball cap.

Slowly, she regains her poise. She goes back to her original two circles. "We use these to show the position on a clock face?" Now she's eager to explain the positions on the clock face. She's back on familiar ground. Before she can show us where 12 o'clock is, the plastic surgeon stands up and thanks her for her time. She's out the door, and we prepare for the next candidate.

"Why did you ask her to draw a breast?" says the radiation oncologist. "To see how observant she is," says the plastic surgeon.

We interview four more candidates. Each time, the radiation oncologist and I wait to see if the plastic surgeon will have the candidate draw a breast. But each interview takes longer than planned; these later candidates are not as practiced in answering questions, and so there is no time at the end for drawing. We have an *n* of one, with no control group, so to speak.

Each candidate has several interviews, and then the interviewers gather in the conference room to rank the day's candidates. I ask the plastic surgeon, "Why did you ask her to draw a breast?"

"To see how observant she is," the plastic surgeon repeats. He goes on, "It's quite common to ask plastic surgery candidates to do something like this."

The radiation oncologist pulls a mechanical pencil out of her white coat pocket. "When I draw a breast, I always draw the heart and lungs," she says.

"The heart and lungs," I say, wonderingly. The plastic surgeon looks surprised as well. I would never think to draw the heart and lungs. They're on the other side of the rib cage from where we do our work as surgeons.

She meticulously draws a cross section of the chest at the level of the breasts, and shows the heart and lungs. She shades in the ribs and muscles that lie between heart, lungs, and breast tissue. I suddenly comprehend how her diagram lets her show a patient how she uses CT scans to guide the radiation treatments, how the radiation beams are precisely programmed to come in tangentially, avoiding the heart and lungs and intersecting in the vicinity of the tumor.

This is how she sees the breast, something to target, lying on top of some important structures that she must spare.

The plastic surgeon takes pen to paper. He draws a graceful breast in silhouette, seen from the side. "The ideal breast," he says, "has a line like this straight to the nipple. The lower pole of the breast is gently curved. The nipple should be at the level of the inframammary fold. As the woman ages, this line curves inward and the nipple droops lower and lower." His breast is the breast of the perfect woman, a breast created by a master sculptor.

Now it is my turn. I draw a breast seen from the front, like a drawing from an anatomy book. I draw the nipple, the areola, the axillary tail. "Here are lobules, here are the ducts," I say. "These lymph nodes drain the breast, these drain the arm." These are all structures that I must consider when I do cancer-directed surgery.

Each of us has drawn our own perspective on the breast. Put our three sketches together and you would still only get an image of the breast, as we see it. Ask a patient to draw a breast, and you might get a completely different perspective—perhaps an infant nursing at a breast. I think of the blind men and the elephant.

Through all of these interviews we have stressed the multidisciplinary nature of breast care. We three—cancer surgeon, plastic surgeon, and radiation oncologist—lead the frontal assault on the tumor. Of course, our breast cancer team relies on many additional specialties—medical oncology, genetics, pathology, diagnostic radiology, social work, nursing, pharmacology, and on and on and on—and perhaps each specialist has a unique view of the breast. What would they draw?

The morning finishes with a lunch for the candidates and the interviewers. I sit next to the young woman, who seems to have fully recovered her aplomb. I talk gently to her, try to reassure her we're not a bad group altogether.

But I'd be willing to bet that somewhere later that night, that nervous young surgeon will be putting pen to paper, trying and trying to draw a breast. I imagine her turning the paper this way and that, maybe even looking up breast drawings on the internet. Practicing, so the next time she gets asked that question, she's ready.

I want to say to her, "There is no one right answer."

---

**CAROL SCOTT-CONNER** is a professor emeritus of surgery at the University of Iowa Carver College of Medicine. She is a founding editor of *The Examined Life Journal*, where she currently serves as fiction editor. In 2023, she received her MFA in narrative medicine from Lenoir-Rhyne University in Hickory, North Carolina.

Her writing explores the space between surgeon and patient, as experienced by a female academic surgeon.

ESSAY

# Top Surgery

ANGELA TANG-TAN

His body opens as if impatient to begin. The skin parts easily, unzipping at the merest touch of the surgeon's scalpel. It's clean, almost bloodless. The subcutaneous vessels burst in tiny scarlet rivulets, which are swallowed in a blink by the suction. The crackle of the Bovie punctuates the tinny pop music playing from the circulator's computer. Smoke wafts upward and I catch the smell of meat, sizzling. Iridescent pearls of fat shimmer and drip under the glare of the overhead lights. I place the skin hooks, catching the razor-sharp points on the edge of the skin. I pull upward and stretch it taut so that the incision gapes wide. My fingers instantly begin to ache.

His breasts blossom into two raw flowers, trumpet-shaped and glistening.

I look down and my breath hitches. Beneath my binder, I feel twin lines of fire sear across my ribcage. It's an echo, a phantom pain, a flinch of anticipation. My body sparks and shivers in recognition.

That morning, at 7:30 AM in the third-floor pre-op, I spot a thin man with a shock of bleach blonde curls and a sparse, dark-haired beard. He sits with his back very straight, in the manner of someone who tends to slouch and is painfully aware of it. He answers the nurse's questions in a voice almost too soft to hear above the din of a dozen other patients in the surrounding beds. His tattooed fingers creep to the strings of his gown, plucking them apart and retying them with quick, birdlike jabs.

*HE/HIM* announces the patient chart.

*Age: 29*

*Sex: Female*

While the nurse does her work, I slip in through the curtains and linger like a ghost with unfinished business. I am a good medical student—I am forever holding my tongue. I never say a word more than I need to. When the nurse leaves, I tell him my name and introduce myself as the medical student rotating through plastic surgery.

"Congratulations on your top surgery," I say. He nods politely.

Then, aghast at my own admission, I add: "Someday I think I might get it too."

It comes out wrong, with a lilt at the end of the sentence, as if it were a question and not a statement. I have never said that before, not here in pre-op, never beneath the harsh fluorescent lights of the hospital at all, and it is as if I hardly know how to form the words on my tongue.

For the first time, his eyes flicker up to meet mine and I glimpse something shy and shining in his gaze.

"Hey," he murmurs. "I'm glad you're here. What are your pronouns?"

I tell him, and what I mean to say is, *It is all right. You can sleep. I know what it's like to look people in the eye and never know what I'll find there. I will not let them call you by the wrong name while you are away. I will do my best to watch over your body until you come home to claim it.*

I draw breath to say something else, I'm not sure what, but we are already out of time.

The resident is here, and the attending with his skin markers. He nods and sheds the chrysalis of his gown. They ask him to stand, sit, raise his arms, lower them. His chest becomes a palimpsest of red, green, and blue. I stand with my back to the wall, drawing silence around me like armor.

---

I take care with the closure. The resident works on the left side, the physician assistant and I on the right. With my right hand, I hold the needle driver between my thumb and ring finger just the way I was taught. With my left hand, I pluck at the edge of the skin with forceps so that I can drive the crescent of the needle into the paper-thin line between dermis and epidermis. It's a running subcuticular suture. *Pierce, pull, pierce, pull.* I've done it many times before, but this time is different. I need to make it perfect. I want to make it beautiful.

Stitch by stitch, I sew the body back together. I weave into each stitch a prayer for healing, a prayer for joy. Slowly, the incision is drawn together by the dissolving suture until the wound becomes invisible. I wipe the incision with a wet cloth and examine the flat expanse of chest, smooth and unencumbered. It is almost as if the skin had never been broken, as if nothing had happened at all.

We place the drains, finish the closure, and stand by as the anesthesiology resident performs the extubation. He announces: "Alright, she's about to wake up. What was her name?"

Someone—an attending anesthesiologist—consults the chart and suggests the deadname.

"The patient uses he/him pronouns," I mutter.

"What?"

"I said, the patient uses he/him pronouns," I say, louder. I give his chosen name.

I have never corrected an attending before, and my tongue is unfamiliar in my mouth. At once, a craven part of me is wishing I had not spoken. I feel that I have careened off the brink of something vast and unforgivable. It is a familiar dread, not unlike when you give an answer to a pimp question and know, before the syllables have left your mouth, that you have gotten it wrong. Suddenly, my binder is suffocating me.

"Oh, okay," says the resident, and he begins to call the patient's name as he stirs. I breathe out. I think of how wrenching it would be, to rise up from the dark lake of anesthesia after top surgery to the cast-off syllables of a deadname.

It happens again as we are wheeling the patient out of the OR. Someone uses his deadname—once, then twice. This time, I do not hesitate when I overhear. I tell them his name and my voice does not waver.

---

It's one of my last days on the plastics rotation and I'm dismissed after PM rounds. I'm lucky—it's only been a twelve-hour day. The hospital is winding down for the weekend. The surgery workroom empties as the day team signs off to the night residents. For a minute, I'm tempted to drive home for a shower and a meal. Instead, my aching feet are drawn in the direction of the post-op recovery unit.

"Hey, I remember you," he breathes as I open the curtains around his bed. His voice is thick with pain and anesthesia. He is alone, and his thin frame is shrouded by a white expanse of bedsheets. The lights in the recovery unit are dimmed, but as I pull the curtains closed again, I realize that he's crying softly. Jewel-bright tears are slicing across his cheek and staining his pillow.

"How's your pain?" I ask.

"Alright. I don't feel much yet."

"May I sit down?"

"Yeah."

I fetch a box of tissues and a warm blanket before pulling up a chair. Then I offer my hand, which he grips in both of his own.

"What's on your mind?"

He exhales a quivering sigh. "This is just . . . so much to process. I can't get the thoughts to quiet down in my head."

"I'm off for the day. I have nowhere else to be for a bit, if you want a little company."

He smiles hesitantly. "Okay. That would be nice."

At first his words come slowly, then faster. Then they pour forth in a great rush, as if they were crowding each other on the way out.

For the next hour, he opens himself to me. He speaks of his girlfriend who lives in Seattle with their two cats, his art exhibition that will open in Europe in September, and his mother who is coming to pick him up from the hospital, who is loving but does not understand. I glimpse the thread of his life, unspooling toward this moment. Behind me, the curtains hold everything else at bay.

Little by little, his breathing eases. Finally, he lets his head fall back on the pillow.

"I should let you rest. You probably won't remember very much of this," I say as I rise to my feet.

"You know, I didn't expect to find someone like me," he whispers, his eyes half closed. "Not here, of all places. I'm glad you were a part of my top surgery. That's important. I want to make sure I remember that."

I reach out and clasp his hand tightly in mine in recognition of the unspoken covenant between us. I imagine our bodies blooming open and folding down into new shapes—better and kinder shapes. And for a moment, I wonder if I have the courage it takes to remake myself, and then the world.

---

**ANGELA TANG-TAN** is a fourth-year medical student at the Keck School of Medicine at the University of Southern California. She graduated from the University of California, Berkeley, in 2020 with a dual degree in neurobiology and psychology before becoming an EMT during the COVID-19 pandemic. She plans to pursue a residency in neurosurgery.

ESSAY

# Beethoven Symphony No. 5

## MITALI CHAUDHARY

I ENTERED THE patient's sunny room, the wide window perfectly framing the city's skyline, and greeted the older gentleman huddled under crisp white sheets. I had already reviewed my notecard encapsulating his medical history, carefully inscribed with medications, to-do lists, and disposition plans. The notecard was shoved deep into my scrubs pocket now, next to twenty-four others—one for each patient under my team—snug against my stethoscope and hastily printed resuscitation guidelines. I wore the shiny new title of Senior Medical Resident awkwardly on my shoulders and, painfully aware of this, was determined to avoid any missteps that might alert someone to my being an imposter.

The patient, blissfully unaware of my internal monologue, fixed his rheumy blue eyes on me and chirped a greeting back. "Advanced vascular dementia," read his notecard. I asked him how his day was and whether he had any medical concerns. The gentleman first shared his opinion on breakfast, then the quality of hospital linens, then moved on to his view on common analgesics. I attempted and reattempted to redirect him to answering my questions about symptomatology, to no avail.

The nape of my neck began to flush warm, and I was alerted to the ticking of my intrinsic timer, now qualifying as weapons-grade from months of honing my time management skills while working in a busy tertiary care center. I thought of the list of patients I had yet to see, the pager that had sliced through the sunlit silence shrilly just moments before, and the junior residents and medical students who would be waiting for me to review plans. The phone in my back pocket was another matter, and the weight of unanswered messages there grew steadily. I began evasive maneuvers, asking directly about my main concerns of pain and bleeding, then pinching the conversation off. His eyes widened, sensing that I would be stepping out soon, and he suddenly proclaimed: "I like Beethoven the best!" I hesitated, suddenly reminded of another me a few years ago who would have delighted in this opportunity to get to know a patient further. "Senior Medical Resident," I heard this version of myself think. I made my excuses and left.

The remainder of the day passed in a flurry of rounds, pages, and shuffled lists crisscrossed with scribbled notes. I thought about that patient while waiting on the homeward-bound subway platform that evening. Guilt filled the pit of my stomach. The idea that I might have made him feel dismissed or unheard gnawed at me. At the same time, I understood that I had responsibilities toward more than one patient now, and that some of the administrative tasks I was involved in were of indirect benefit to him as well.

But how does one communicate this to a patient in such a small wedge of time constrained by other competing wedges? Was this how it would always be now that I was no longer a junior learner who had more freedom to explore and take gratification in the individuality of those I cared for?

I didn't like that thought. It had not fully occurred to me how much it meant to be invited into patients' lives and how much it added to my day.

As I puzzled over this, the ruby red columns and tiles of the subway station refocused into view. I took in the speckled stone floors, the warm exhalations of the tunnels, and the grimy tracks that anchored the scene in front of me. I realized I had made my way to the station nearest my former high school, where I had spent time immemorial waiting—for friends, for parents to pick me up, for the train to my job. I was reminded of the geriatrics unit where I had volunteered through my late teens. Memories materialized of providing warm blankets, holding weathered hands, and being an avid audience to patients with delirium. I smiled inwardly at the feeling of satisfaction that came along with those memories and found myself yearning for it.

I returned to work the next day with an updated to-do list. Among the reminders of discharge summaries and referrals to send, I had listed "Beethoven." I strode to the patient's room in the midmorning, determined. Again, I found him sitting there, blinking against beams of sunlight in a pile of blankets. I asked about pain and bleeding—and then I asked about his taste in music. He smiled widely and invoked the composer once again, relating a patchwork of detail about his life and work. I then asked what his favorite piece was. He watched me enter his quick reply into my phone's internet browser. We looked idly out at the cityscape, listening to the first commanding notes of Symphony No. 5 float out of the speaker held between us. In time, he turned his wide smile back to me.

---

**MITALI CHAUDHARY** is a third-year resident in internal medicine at the University of Toronto. Her interests include research on the intersection of teaching and advocacy, and hunting for the best almond croissant in the city.

ESSAY

# Beholding Something Fine

## LAURA JOHNSRUDE

We lingered in the corner of a delivery room while the obstetrics staff attended to a laboring woman. The soon-to-be-mother was writhing and moaning, clenching and stretching, with the otherworldly work of it all. She transformed, suddenly, moving from supine arching to standing straight up in the stirrups, like an angry Greek goddess, bellowing her pain.

She was not our patient, though. We were waiting for the baby.

We, pediatricians-in-training in the late 1980s, had been paged to attend the high-risk birth. Maybe the baby was premature with a risk of respiratory distress due to immature lungs. Maybe the mother was addicted to opiates, so the baby was exposed too. Maybe the mother's water broke more than twenty-four hours ago, so the baby was at risk of infection. Or twins were expected. Or the baby's heartbeat was erratic. Or there wasn't enough fluid around the baby. Or the mother had had no prenatal care at all.

Standing by the infant bed and warmer, I watched the large-bellied woman crouch, then unfold her knees and back, rising up toward the ceiling, untethered, unhinged. She was on drugs, word was, and we, the pediatricians-in-training, readied our resuscitation equipment.

We each poked a single hole into our paper facial masks and threaded a clear plastic tube through the tear into our mouths, biting it between our teeth. The other end of the straw between our lips was connected to a clear plastic container—a DeLee Mucus Trap—with its second clear plastic tube dangling toward the floor. We stood there, two of us, awaiting the stressed newborn, who may have already passed meconium—the first stool—and may have some of the sticky stuff inside their mouth. We, the pediatricians-in-training, were there to suck it out and catch it in the DeLee canister, the snare between baby and us.

It's said that in the past, doctors just sucked the green slime directly into their own mouths and spat it out.

The nurses coaxed the gravid woman down to deliver, but the image hung there, for me, even years later, after I'd writhed and moaned and clenched and stretched and birthed my own children. The laboring woman, her face upturned, beholding something fine, or something terrible, her bare feet in the metal stirrups, the whole of her balanced there in the air, roaring.

We, the pediatricians-in-training, wanted the baby to not breathe for just a few seconds, to pause for our ministrations. The obstetrician would hand off the child to us right away, and we would thread the distal dangling DeLee tubing into the baby's slack, open mouth—don't breathe, don't breathe—and suck on the tubing we held between our teeth, while dipping that other end around the gums and tongue of the just-born, vacuuming the green slime into the DeLee trap—quickly, quickly—hoping to prevent meconium aspiration into the infant's lungs with its first deep breath.

We'd jostle the newborn then, after clearing the mouth, wanting the limp one to stretch and startle now, take a big gulp of air now. Under the warmer. Wanting the face to pink up, under the lights. Wanting the limp one to breathe, breathe.

Your turn, now, take a breath.

Cry, little one. She needs to hear you cry.

---

**LAURA JOHNSRUDE** is a retired pediatrician living in Louisville, Kentucky. Her essays have appeared in *Fourth Genre, Bellevue*

*Literary Review, River Teeth, Hippocampus, Brevity, Appalachian Review, The Spectacle, Please See Me, Minerva Rising, Drunk Monkeys, Under the Gum Tree, The Examined Life Journal, Sweet, Swing,* and in *The Boom Project* anthology. "Beholding Something Fine" was nominated for a Pushcart Prize.

ESSAY

# Stroppy Sevens

TRISHA PAUL

*What do you want?*
 Your leery question greets me. Every morning, without fail.
 "I'm just saying hi," I say calmly, as I do every day.
 Your gaze quickly returns to the TV screen.
 From across the room, I watch you for a moment. There you are, comfortable in your near-nakedness, nothing on but a diaper. As you sit cross-legged, your shoulders slouch forward, your face inches from the screen. With your head craned upward, your dark eyes peer out from underneath your disheveled black hair, fixed keenly on the TV.
 *Feral.* Never before have I heard such an ugly word describe a child so young. They warned me about you. How you crawl on tables, hissing and growling. Choking yourself when things don't go your way. Don't let him get too close, they said, for you have discovered the pain that pinching above the elbow elicits.
 You are the child who scares me.
 Nevertheless, today is different. As I wait expectantly for your mundane greeting and brief glance, your dark eyes instead hold my gaze. Your legs unfold from under you, and you hop out of the chair.
 You're walking straight at me. You waddle, shifting the weight of your pudgy body, from one leg to the next. Right, left, right, left. Back and forth you go, your pace quickening as you move toward

me. There's mischief in your dry, chapped lips, your crooked baby teeth peering out from a lopsided smile (or is that a glimmer of a snarl?).

You are getting closer. I find my body inching away from your approach, taking one step backward. I try to steady myself, channeling all the confidence that I do not have to stand up straight, although my shoulders creep up unapologetically. My heart roars. My mind darts in an attempt to escape the fear I feel throughout my entire body. I brace myself for what is to come, feeling my core tighten. Unsure, I am immobilized by uncertainty.

And there I stand as you hug me, your arms wrapping tightly around my middle. "You're so skinny," you say to me.

I stand there, within your embrace, mesmerized by this moment. My eyes are wet, my mouth dry. My knees unbuckle as my muscles relax, my heart softening. My mind wanders, wondering how such a sweet boy can be turned into such a troubled soul. Troubled by my own instincts, my own repulsion, my own wariness of you, you who are no more than seven years old.

Slowly, one before the other, I wrap my arms around you, and sigh.

---

**TRISHA PAUL** is a pediatric oncologist and palliative care physician, a narrative medicine scholar, and a writer. She holds an MFA in creative nonfiction writing from New York University and her writing appears in anthologies and medical journals such as *JAMA*. "Stroppy Sevens" was nominated for a Pushcart Prize. Paul loves caring for her Little Free Library, dancing barefoot, and collecting anything made of cork.

# Acknowledgments

While looking back at the fine work published in *Intima* since its inception in 2011, I'm filled with gratitude for my fellow editors, who've contributed their time and energy to finding the finest stories, essays, and poems that we now showcase in *Where It Hurts*. I'm overwhelmed by the generosity of spirit and amount of free time each of them gave to our mission of lifting up new voices in the medical humanities. Each demonstrated true commitment, showing up to make it happen twice a year, year after year.

When the stars align, good work happens, as do miracle connections. I thank my lucky stars for my agent, Laurie Fox of the Linda Chester Literary Agency, for her years of support, guidance, inspiration, and friendship. As the singer Laura Nyro wrote, you "ornament the world" for me and everyone you know. I want to honor the agency's legendary founder, Linda Chester, and acknowledge the inspiring agents Darlene Chan and D. Patrick Miller as well.

I'd especially like to thank Sara Zatopek at The Experiment, who, as my editor, holds a special place of honor in this project. From the beginning, Sara brought her keen intelligence, perceptive close reading, and deep appreciation for the original voices and complex narratives in the book. Our editorial board thanks the publisher, Matthew Lore, cofounder and president of The Experiment, for his curiosity, interest, and support of the work we do. We also thank Beth Bugler, who designed the cover and selected the cover art from a series of oil paintings titled "The Student's White Coat" by Mohamed Mahfouz Sylla, published in the Spring 2022 issue of *Intima*; Zach Pace (what a perfect name for the role as managing editor) for the coordination and attention to details that make a book come together on time; and Ann J. Kirschner, the copy editor, who paid careful attention to our words and punctuation. Thank you to photographer Kyle Ericksen for my portrait.

Of course, neither *Intima* nor this book would have existed without Rita Charon, who led the team of brilliant dreamers at Columbia University to establish the field of narrative medicine. The founders of *Intima*—graduate students in the first class of Columbia's Narrative Medicine Master of Science degree program—were Jennifer Adaeze Okwerekwu, Shawna Benston, Dana Gage, Sneha Mantri, Jase Miles-Perez, Jesús Rivera, and Mario de la Cruz. After receiving a postgraduate fellowship from Columbia to redesign and rethink the journal, I was fortunate to have Cindy Smalletz as a tireless and intelligent adviser, who not only understood the content of theintima.org but also had the technical brilliance to help me build a site worthy of its mission.

I'm grateful for everyone who has been on our editorial board through the years: Priya Amin, Saljooq M. Asif, Anjana Bala, Timothy J. Barreiro, Maida Broudo, Bruce H. Campbell, Ruth Marks Case, Lala Tanmoy Das, Olivia Davies, Roxana Delbene, Nelly Edmondson, Joseph Eveld, Sina Foroutanjazi, Malini Gandhi, Maureen Hirthler, Aubrie-Ann Jones, Zahra H. Khan, Sara Kohrt, Vivian Lam, Elizabeth Lanphier, Zohar Lederman, Jennifer Li, Sophia Li, Priscilla Mainardi, Eve Makoff, Natasha Massoudi, Bonnie McDougall Olson, Trisha Paul, Rachel Prince, Angelica Recierdo, Holly Schechter, Michael Smolka, Elizabeth Spradley, Brandon Sultan, Amir Tarsha, Daly Walker, Annie Xiao, and Grace Yi. I also applaud those who contributed: Elena DeBre, Andrew Flynn, Anita Hill, Nina Molina, and Joanna Sommer.

Each person brought talent, energy, and unique abilities to the editorial table (even though we never actually sat together at any table or in any room). We read through thousands of submissions, voiced our opinions in notes, and cast our votes via Submittable, a publishing platform that was a godsend for a fledgling administrator dizzy with keeping tabs on submissions as the numbers grew from twenty to seventy-five to over five hundred.

I'd like to single out Mario de la Cruz, a founding editor who remains active as an editor and creative director. His clear vision, impressive big-picture views, and decisive opinions are invaluable when making tough calls about what to accept and what to decline. Mario is *Intima*'s guiding light, and his wisdom and brilliance have made the journal a place where empathy and intelligence come together in the most satisfying ways.

As managing editor for many years, Maureen Hirthler steadied the ship during the late nights and rocky reviews; Bruce Campbell stepped into that role in 2024 and connects our far-flung group in Zoom meetings, book reviews, and our Crossroad blogs. Longtime editors Angelica, Priscilla, Daly, Holly, Joe, Brandon, and Trisha continue to have profound impact on the work we publish. To all of our editors, especially those who have just joined the team, I send my deep appreciation for their support and impressive skills.

How would I exist without my friends? Pamela, Andrew, Susan, the Moms—Joyce, Debbie, Marcella, and Sarah—Aline, Anne, Jill, Marilyn, Lauren, Maryellen, Annette, Molly, Lisa, Ross, Jack, Gina and Scott, Jane and Adam, Gloria-Jean and Nat, DeLora and Michael, Polly and Rex, Nancy, Claudy, Farrah, Patrick, Tim, Judy, the two Dons, Mindy, Ellie, the Mermaids—Linda and Susanna—the Davids, the Book Club, Keith, Allegra, Marlene, Derek, Maria, Nina, Cindy, Hal, Tara, Laurie, Evan, and Kris. I love you all.

I thank editors Debi Dunn, Dale Hrabi, Michael Miller, Janice Min, Martha Nelson, Charla Lawhon, Shaye Areheart, and Allison Gwinn, who've taught me the subtleties of my craft. To Anita Bethel, On-ke Wilde, and Betsy Miller: The light in the world dimmed when you left us, but my memory of you burns bright.

These friends are all family to me, but my family reigns supreme: my beautiful sisters Katherine and Gloria and their wonderful families. The Vlcek clan: I love you! I know my parents, Dorothy and Fred, watch over all of us with love and pride. I know they would be proud of all of us. My darling Roy, his wife Andrea, and their daughter, Veradonna, bring me infinite joy.

And to my husband, Dana: Your daily presence feels like heaven on earth to me.

# About the Editor

DONNA BULSECO is a journalist and editor who holds graduate degrees in English from Brown University and in narrative medicine from Columbia University. Through the years, she has published work in *The New York Times*, *Wall Street Journal*, *InStyle*, *Self*, and *The Purist*. As editor-in-chief of *Intima: A Journal of Narrative Medicine*, she works with an editorial board of clinicians, educators, and writers, who review and select from over one thousand submissions a year to produce the journal. She lives with her husband, the musician and producer Dana Vlcek, in New York City.

**theintima.org | ⊚intimajournal**